eco-eating

a guide to
balanced eating
for health &

vitality

Vickie H Heather
7/15/02

sapoty brook

Lothian
B O O K S

Thomas C. Lothian Pty Ltd
11 Munro Street, Port Melbourne, Victoria 3207

National Library of Australia
Cataloguing-in-Publication data:

Brook, Sapoty.
   Eco-eating.

   Bibliography.
   Includes index.
   ISBN 0 85091 736 0.

   1. Food habits. 2 Nutrition – Psychological aspects.
   I. Title.

615.854

Cover design by Modern Art Production Group
Text design by Tom Kurema
Illustrations by Ciska Cassa
Diagrams by Sapoty Brook; chart redrawn by Pages in
Action
Printed in Australia by Griffin Paperbacks

Foreword

S apoty Brook has provided us with a beautifully succinct and witty book, full of practical and accessible nutritional information.

Food as medicine, visual information presented in chart form, insights into mineral balancing, and other revolutionary ideas abound. Minerals are the basis of our cellular physiology, and Sapoty Brook gives us an elegant yet simple means to direct them to our advantage.

The name of the game is eco-eating, tuning into our bodies' needs and satisfying them with minimum stress to ourselves and the planet.

The young and old are given specific advice, while adults are encouraged to cut loose from the tyranny of the kitchen and enjoy the leisurely life of the Symbiotic. For some this may be a way of life, for others a chance to explore a new approach to eating in order to clean out and rebalance themselves.

In this age of chronic degenerative diseases, Sapoty gives us the means to set the scene for prevention or recovery.

At last here is a book that stands out from the burgeoning literature on nutrition like a poppy in a pasture.

Dr Jamie Duff
MD (MBChB, BSc)

Contents

Foreword by Dr Jamie Duff   iii
Why Read This Book?   vi
Introduction   1
'Mangoes', by Richard Tipping   4

PART 1   **THE SYMBIOTIC WAY**   5

A Fruitful Journey   7
What Does It All Mean?   15
Eating for: The Past   29
             Evolution of Consciousness   31
             Bones and Soft Tissue Health   36
             Body Fluids Health   45
             Energy   49
             Digestion   51
             Vitamins and Minerals   60
             Immunity   65
             The Heart   71
             The Teeth   73
             Weight Loss   74
             Weight Gain   79
             Cooling   82
             Warmth   84
             Longevity   86
             The Climate   91
             The Seasons   93
             The Spirit   95
             Happiness   97

CONTENTS

Pleasure 100
Cravings 103
Addictions 105
Travelling 107
Sunshine 109
Beauty 111
Elegance 113
Peace 115
Satisfaction 117
Money 119
Time 120
Sleep 121
Work 123
Action 125
Sport 126
Thought 129
Emotions 130
Personality 133
Sex 135
Children 137
Getting High 140
The Environment 141
A New Society 144
The Future 146
Love 148

PART 2   **WHAT TO EAT?** 149

Recipes 151
The CaPNaK Chart in Detail 160
Food Composition Data 170
Epilogue 177
References 178
Index 181
Questionnaire 185
Training Consultation 186
Order a CaPNaK Chart Colour Poster 186

v

Why read this book?

You are probably scanning bookshelves on health right now, maybe looking for a book that will give you a new perspective, an insight into new dimensions of health. Perhaps you want to reach higher levels of holistic health in connection with the planet Earth.

This book will help you do just that. It is an original synthesis of ideas; it is groundbreaking information for a new way of living. I hope this book will help you improve your life and our environment.

The theories and advice presented here are based on my own study and experience. Consult your preferred medical authority before changing to this eating system; particular caution should be exercised with children, the elderly and frail, and by pregnant women. Vitamin and mineral supplementation may be necessary in some cases.

Acknowledgements

I wish to acknowledge the teaching, assistance and advice provided by my father, Dr Peter Crooke (medical practitioner); my mother, Judith Crooke (counsellor); Amanda Cartwright (naturopath); Linda Grierson (nurse); Dr Jamie Duff (medical practitioner); and all my friends who read the draft manuscript.

Five per cent of the author's net profits from the sale of this book will be donated to environmental organisations.

Sapoty Brook, MSc

Introduction

Awareness of a vast new world of nutrition is spreading to the corners of the world. Everywhere people of good will are struggling to implement new practices and principles. Soon a long-forgotten nutritional territory will provide a fertile basis for the renewal of the being that is human.

A map of this new world of nutrition, the CaPNaK Chart* (pronounced 'Cap-nack') is given on page 166. In the past a few explorers have sailed into the realm of CaPNaK. Some recorded incredible experiences of healing, vitality and agelessness.

A tiny band of puritans, the Symbiotics, travelled large distances across CaPNaK to set up a colony in the realm of fruit. They have formed subgroups, known as the Fruitarians and the Live Fooders. Many of the Symbiotics have established trade routes from the land of fruit to the land of green-leaf vegetables and the land of nuts and seeds.

A dark cloud of confusion and conflict threatens this hopeful land of juice and freshness. There is a territorial dispute between two major ideological forces: the Symbiotics and the Macrobiotics. (Symbiotic means 'harmonious life', Macrobiotics 'whole or long life.')

Based on the strong traditions of ancient cultures the Macrobiotics are firmly established in a position of power. They have a formidable cuisine based on rice and other cereals, but spurn fruit. Various influential splinter groups have formed, such as the Standard Macrobiotics, Pritikins, Vegetarians and Vegans.

---

* A chart showing how to balance the four major minerals in your food: calcium (Ca), phosphorus (P), sodium (Na) and potassium (K).

These groups have demonstrated such potent benefits of their nutritional ideology that government health organisations are creating regulations to convert heartburn to heartbeat: heart disease is being reduced through government nutritional policies.

Unfortunately there is a wide ideological ocean between the Macrobiotics and the Symbiotics because of the digestive incompatibility of fruits and cereals. Brewers have known for millenia about combining cereals and sugary substances. This results in a fermenting gaseous fluid that can turn the most poised human into a rather drunk one. When this kind of bacterial fermentation occurs excessively in the body it produces some rather unpleasant sensations and odours. So the Macrobiotics have rejected fruit, and labelled it an unbalanced food, not to be taken as a contender for contemporary mainstream eating.

The now-powerful Macrobiotics so derided the Symbiotics that they became almost extinct. But the Symbiotics have recently been quietly organising themselves into an international support group, called the Fruitarian Network. The Fruitarian Network is co-ordinated from that land of freedom and cultural diversity known as Australia.*

By occupying the fringe regions of the CaPNaK Chart, the Macrobiotics have surrounded the Symbiotics. Using such unbalancing cuisine as seaweed, miso and beans, as well as their staple cereals, they swing across CaPNaK with gleeful abandonment. They often navigate as if in a one-dimensional realm, with only the complementary directions of yin and yang. This one-dimensional navigation can lead to confusion of locations in the two-dimensional land of CaPNaK. Some Macrobiotics have pointed out the importance of using the acid–alkaline dimension as well as that of yin-yang (Aihara 1982).

Despite such positive steps, the ideological ocean between the Macrobiotics and the Symbiotics remains. This book is a guide for those who wish to explore the realm of CaPNaK. I am a Symbiotic leaning towards a scientific approach to the subject, and I do not

---

* Fruitarian Network, PO Box 293, Trinity Beach, Qld 4879.

remain exclusively in the land of fruit. Above all, I emphasise the experiential; this is a work of synthesis, rather than analysis.

The CaPNaK Chart was born out of conflict and into controversy. It expresses the basic schism between civilisation and nature. Should we base our diet on cereals, which have been the nutritional basis of civilisation? Should we base our diet on fruits, which are the natural food of primates, including pre-civilised humankind? Is a truly natural civilisation possible where we combine the benefits of civilised life with a natural symbiotic relationship with our food and our planet?

This book takes a step towards resolving these questions. The CaPNaK Chart provides a new and more rigorous way of relating the physical and mental effects of the four most prevalent food minerals: calcium, phosphorus, sodium and potassium. The locations of food on the chart have been calculated from food composition data (see pages 170–6), and equations (see page 169) to provide a more meaningful framework that takes account of the primary roles of these minerals in physiology. The chart encourages the use of whole foods, rather than mineral supplements, to provide the mineral balance.

Mangoes

mangoes are not cigarettes
mangoes are fleshy skinful passionate fruits
mangoes are hungry to be sucked
mangoes are glad to be stuck in the teeth
mangoes like slush & kissing

mangoes are not filter tipped
mangoes are idiosyncratic seasonal seducers
mangoes are worse than adams apple
mangoes are what parents & parliaments warn against
mangoes like making rude noises

mangoes are not extra mild
mangoes are greedy delicious tongueteasers
mangoes are violently soft
mangoes are fibrous intestinal lovebites
mangoes like beginning once again

mangoes are not cigarettes
mangoes are tangible sensual intelligence
mangoes are debauched antisocialites
mangoes are a positive good in the world
mangoes like poetry

Richard Tipping

Reprinted from Richard Tipping, *Domestic Hardcore*, University of Queensland Press, 1975, with the author's permission.

1

The
Symbiotic
Way

A Fruitful Journey

S it back. Relax. Imagine yourself in the future. You feel fundamentally different. You are filled with a wonderful energetic feeling. You feel even more vitality than when you were a teenager. Your body is slim and firm, and your skin is clear. Your hair gleams, and your eyes sparkle. You are intensely alive!

Your ailments have been swept away and your body is so vital that ordinary sickness or infections are masterfully defeated by your immune system. You can maintain steady physical and mental activity all day with a stable level of energy. Your mood is calm and tranquil, and you feel light and full of good humour. Reaching toward the fruit bowl for a mango, you smile with happiness.

Regrettably, most of us never have this experience. Most of us live with some imbalance, disorder or disease. I long for a world where everyone lives in health and happiness, but there are a myriad of forces that lead to suffering. We all try to reach a better balance within our perception of the constraints of our capabilities and opportunities. New avenues of opportunity sometimes open to us, and suddenly we find we have hidden potentialities that we didn't know existed.

Such was my experience with nutrition. I will tell you my story, but first let me warn you that it is a chronicle of setbacks. Nevertheless, it is also a chronicle of solutions: solutions that have worked and led me to vibrant health.

I began life with a few setbacks in my health. At a very young age I developed a mild hearing loss due to deterioration of some nerves in my inner ears. One kidney began to malfunction, and was removed when I was five years old. Fortunately, because I was so young my other kidney grew larger, and took over the work of my missing kidney. Without such basic setbacks I may never have developed my regard for health. With the care of loving parents I adjusted to these conditions and eventually did well enough at school to enter university. I studied hard for degrees in science and engineering, and ambitiously entered the workforce.

However, I certainly was not healthy. My years of dedication to study and inattention to my health had kept me thin and unwell. I was a pale and pimply young man who caught every cold and flu that passed by. I was addicted to sweets and coffee for enough energy to work. Occasionally people would comment that I looked 'like death warmed up'!

I travelled through South-East Asia, where I picked up a nasty staphylococcus infection that took two years and many courses of antibiotics to expel. This infection convinced me of the importance of the immune system and the relative impotence of medicine. I realised that I must take full responsibility for my health. Some friends also encouraged me to take up jogging.

I began to take more interest in developing a scientific understanding of health. I already had some very real knowledge of health problems in a developed country. My father was a doctor, and as a child I saw him go out, night after night, to heart-attack victims. I remember seeing drug advertisements with glossy pictures of cholesterol deposits in arteries, and I had asked him whether, if people stopped eating so much cholesterol, they would stop getting heart attacks. He was not sure; there was no definitive evidence at the time.

With more scientific training and some success as an engineer, I was now willing to explore beyond the horizons of consensus science (those theories that the vast majority of scientific thinkers consider correct models of reality). I knew that interest in nutrition was rapidly growing, undermining the conventional wisdom of medical practitioners. I thought the study of nutrition might be the missing piece in the health puzzle.

I read a few popular nutrition books, such as Frances Lappe's *Diet for a Small Planet* (1975), and became convinced that a cereal-based diet was healthier than a meat-and-dairy-product-based diet. It seemed to me that with its low cholesterol and fat, a grain-based diet was at least a partial preventative against heart failure and other cardiovascular diseases. Research also correlated certain forms of cancer with meat eating. I substantially reduced my intake of meat and dairy foods and increased the amount of grains. I weaned myself off sugar and caffeine too, despite considerable withdrawal symptoms, such as headaches. With such incremental changes in my eating behaviour, gradually my health improved.

This success whetted my appetite for better health. I wondered what the limit was to this potential for health. I had heard and read about the benefits of meditation, so I tried it, and found an immediate relief from stress. I was working in a high-pressure, internationally-mobile, high-technology job, and living a fast, inner-city social life. In my spare time I was also struggling over an invention for which I later won an Australian Inventors' Award. I was very stressed. Through the meditation my awareness expanded, and my mental and emotional stability deepened rapidly. Meditation provided a basis for me to conduct more profound experimentation and exploration of potential for good health in particular.

Two years later, in search of wider horizons, I left my job as an engineer, and joined the University of Western Australia as a research scientist. One day in 1981 I came across a book in the university bookshop called *The Health Revolution* by Ross Horne. Flipping through the pages I saw that this book contained information I had been looking for about the relationships between nutrition and disease. It revealed an impressively detailed and holistic understanding of health, focusing primarily on nutrition and exercise. It recommended a diet of mostly fruit, with a minimum of cooked foods. The objective was to maximise enzyme content and reduce the biochemical destruction of food occurring during cooking. I took up jogging for half an hour every morning, and began eating kilos of fresh fruit and vegies. My friends commented on the dramatic improvement in my health. Within a few months my acne dried up, and my skin became clear and smooth.

I still found myself craving for and eating some cooked cereal products, such as bread. However, my reading convinced me that cooked grains were not an optimal food, mainly because of the destruction of food enzymes in cooking. According to *The Health*

Revolution, this enzyme deficiency results in the overloading of the pancreas during the digestion of cooked cereals.

Curious to get an objective assessment of my fitness, I took a fitness test at the university's gym. When I finished I was astounded to hear the instructor congratulate me, saying I was the fittest person in my age group they had tested all year. He went on to tell me I was the third-fittest person in all age groups! I was twenty-eight at the time.

Eating mostly fruit was a delightful experience. I also ate some vegetables, nuts, seeds and sprouted grain. Books, such as *Survival into the 21st Century* (1975) by Viktoras Kulvinskas, guided and inspired me.

However, not everything was going smoothly: my digestion fluctuated between constipation and diarrhoea. I became a hazard of noxious gases, which any EPA emissions control officer would put off the road instantly. Thinking back, I am horrified at what my friends endured! Over the following three years my intestines became increasingly chaotic, and finally I succumbed to a couple of opportunistic intestinal infections. I tried fasting briefly, but by that time I was underweight so in desperation I took a single-dose antibiotic. Within twenty-four hours I was gulping down avocados and recovering rapidly.

Out of the darkness of this setback was to rise a new dawn. I was still eating sprouted grain and nuts. I began to suspect that the water used for sprouting carried the bacterium and virus that had infected me. This was the final spur that I needed to try not eating cereals. I took a quantum leap into fruit.

Revelation! My chaotic digestion smoothed out in three days, and became a sublime supersonic experience of intestinal enlightenment! By eating raw fruit and vegetables, I found myself transported to a realm of digestive bliss!

Viktoras Kulvinskas was right! Cereals are unnecessary, even deleterious, and should not be eaten with fruit. Maybe the myth of pure fruitarianism is also a reality, I thought. I experimented with eating only fruit, and for many months found it a viable way of eating.

However, after almost a year my gums became more sensitive, some tooth decay set in, I had cramp more often, and I found I craved salty foods. I had thought that if I was to have any trouble as a pure fruitarian it would relate to minerals, especially sodium and calcium. I had disliked milk as a child, and suspected that my body might be low in calcium. Nutritional references indicated that gum sensitivity, pyorrhoea, tooth decay and cramp are often indicative of a calcium deficiency.

Kulvinskas had mentioned that calcium deficiency is also related to acidity of the body resulting from an acidic diet. I knew that meat, cereals and nuts contain an abundance of phosphorus, which forms acidic compounds. I began to consider that my years of eating such acid-forming foods and Spartan eating of foods containing calcium had left me with a marginal calcium deficiency. This condition is very common (especially among post-menopausal women).

So, when these symptoms appeared, I decided to reintroduce eating green-leaf vegetables, which are a good source of sodium and calcium. I became a herbo-fruitarian. It was time for me to make a more thorough investigation of the mineral content of various foods.

The macrobiotic diet places great emphasis on the sodium–potassium balance in food. This concept of balance led me to wonder whether calcium was subject to balance in a similar way. Such thoughts led me to consider that a calcium–phosphorus balance could also be a useful concept of nutritional balance. I envisaged a system of macrobiotic balance using mostly raw (living) foods, which Macrobiotics had so assiduously shunned.

The CaPNaK Chart

For a year I pondered how the mineral content of foods could be displayed in a useful way. The effect of each food on the mineral balance of the body was the crucial factor to express. Eventually, I realised that by subtracting the balancing ratios of minerals from the total mineral content, the residual quantity of minerals expressed the residual impact on the body. Thus, I developed the Ca (calcium)–P (phosphorus)–Na (sodium)–K (potassium) or CaPNaK Chart.

I put the first CaPNaK Chart together in early 1988 on a laptop computer. It was difficult to interpret because it was based on milligrams of minerals per Calorie (4 kilojoules) of food. However, I became familiar with it, and used it continually.

It was like wandering around in a dark room, and then finding the light switch. Suddenly a whole new dimension of clarity and control of my physical and mental states became available to me. I found I could end various occasional physical annoyances that many people take for granted, such as muscle cramps, dizzy spells, constipation, fatigue, headache, indigestion, coldness, hotness, insomnia, restlessness, and even toothache. Many more benefits of the CaPNaK approach became clear, and led me to refine the CaPNaK Chart and write this book.

As if to reaffirm the importance of calcium balance, a few months later someone fell on me, cracking my rib. I decided to get a bone mineral density scan, and found that my bone mineral density was 20 per cent below the average for my age. So I increased my intake of green-leaf vegetables to about 750 g a day; more recently, on the advice of a naturopath, I have supplemented my diet each day with calcium hydroxyl apatite tablets, which provided me with 500 mg of elemental calcium. These tablets are made from powdered bone, and are acceptable to me since I am not strictly vegan. My tooth and bone problems have now disappeared, and I enjoy superb health.

One of the immediate benefits to me of the CaPNaK Chart was its clear distinction between acid-forming and alkali-forming foods. By preferentially eating alkali-forming food, I have gradually reduced my acidity. The increased alkalinity of my body-mind* has enabled me to retain more body fat. As a result, after being too thin my whole life, over the past few years my weight has finally increased to a satisfactory level. You can read about weight control using the CaPNaK Chart in a later chapter.

---

* 'Mindbody' usually refers to the relations between mind and body (e.g. 'the mind-body problem' of philosophy). 'Body-mind' (as used here) refers to the mind and body as a dyad or integrated whole entity.

The Fruitarian Network

In 1988, soon after I completed the first CaPNaK Chart, I was invited to speak at a meeting of the Australian Natural Health Society in a suburb of Sydney. There were several people present who were enthusiastic about the idea of setting up a support group for fruit-eating people. Those who oriented their eating primarily around fruit, rather than cereal, needed their own organisation. We subsequently held a meeting, and founded the Fruitarian Network. The network is a support group for those people who eat fruit as their primary, but not necessarily sole, source of food.

As a result of the growing demand for information on this eating lifestyle and the dedicated co-ordination of Rene Beresford, the network has grown. At present the network has about 325 members. The *Fruitarian Network News* is published quarterly. Many members express their views and experiences of fruitarianism through the newsletter, and it is providing a practical forum worldwide for debate and support.

At present the *Fruitarian Network News* remains biased towards pure fruitarian idealism. Much has been published on fruitarianism, but we must remain alert for inexperienced zealous fruitarian authors promoting overly idealistic views and extremist practices. In particular, the fruitarian scene is plagued by the belief that all disease is caused solely by toxins in the body-mind. This results in an emphasis on elimination of toxins, and fasting *ad nauseam*, and blinds the believer to serious consideration of nutritional deficiencies and infections.

Vitamin B_{12}

For nine years I ate virtually no meat or dairy foods. At one of my regular blood tests, to my surprise I learnt that I had become a little low in vitamin B_{12}. I had hoped that my intestinal bacteria would spare me this indignity by synthesising B_{12}.

Not wanting to take any risks of nerve damage I immediately had some vitamin B_{12} injections. Again I confronted another decision. Would I supplement this with B_{12} tablets, or eat a processed food such as tempeh (a vegan source of B_{12}), or eat a little raw fish? Nature as it is, or nature how we would like it to be? I opted for nature as it is, with a little raw fish, about 100 g a week, to be precise. My vitamin B_{12} and related iron levels have soared.

If our fruit and vegetables were coming from the forest, they would be full of juicy insects and grubs, and covered with bacteria, all packed with B_{12}. It would not be necessary to resort to eating higher beings such as fish. Until then, I remain a herbo-pisco-fruitarian. I apologise for not including any grasshoppers on the CaPNaK Chart! There is always scope for improvement; isn't there?

Once we pass our prime in life, optimum health can only be defined as the slowest rate of deterioration. Improvements in nutrition and lifestyle can bring about improvements in health, but eventually deterioration returns. I cannot say what deterioration my journey has in store for me, but with a little luck and a lot of care it will happen slowly. Meanwhile, the control and balance of the states of body-mind achievable with the CaPNaK eating system enhance the quality of my life. It can do the same for you.

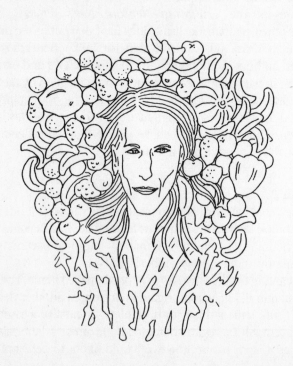

What Does It All Mean?

T he first question I expect to hear when someone sees the CaPNaK Chart is 'What does it all mean?' It is about achieving higher levels of health, and reaching optimum performance in whatever you do. It empowers you to balance and control states of your body and mind.

Here is a miniature diagram of the CaPNaK Chart; the detailed chart showing the locations of individual foods is on page 166.

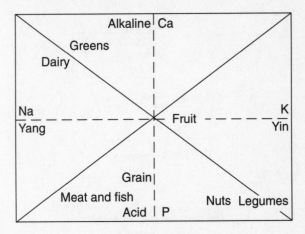

The CaPNaK Chart.

Obviously, the positions of the foods on the chart have significance. Look closely at the background. There are four triangles meeting at a single point, like looking down on a pyramid from above. Maybe the ancient Egyptians knew; it's all to do with complementary balance. I call the single meeting point the balance point.

15

To understand the significance of this balancing and the location of the food groups, look at the chart in parts. The dotted line going from left to right is the sodium–potassium axis:

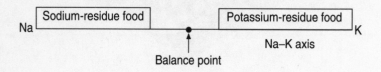

The sodium–potassium axis.

Foods higher in sodium-residue are further to the left; foods higher in potassium-residue are further to the right.

The dotted line going from the bottom to the top of the CaPNaK Chart is the phosphorus–calcium axis, shown left to right here:

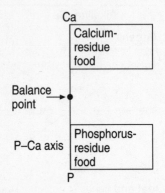

The phosphorus–calcium axis.

Foods higher in calcium-residue are closer to the top; foods higher in phosphorus-residue are closer to the bottom.

Every food has a residue on both the sodium–potassium axis and the phosphorus–calcium axis. Combining the axes at right angles to each other on a surface gives a complete representation of the residues, and the possibility of balancing in both dimensions independently.

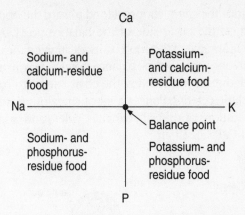

Mineral residues in each quadrant of the CaPNaK Chart.

Look at the location of greens on the CaPNaK Chart. You should now be able to work out that they are sodium- and calcium-residue foods.

Imagine holding up a finger. Balance the CaPNaK Chart on your fingertip, at the balance point where the triangles meet. Now choose a food on the chart. Imagine that as you eat this food you are placing this food on its location on the chart. The chart will tilt down on that side of the balance point.

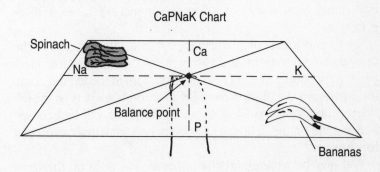

Balance of complementary foods: spinach is a calcium (Ca)- and sodium (Na)-residue food, banana a phosphorus (P)- and potassium (K)-residue food.

To rebalance the chart, choose a food toward the opposite edge of the chart on the other side of the balance point. As you eat, imagine placing some of this food on its location on the chart. If the first food is a long way from the balance point, you will only need to eat a little of the second to bring the chart back into balance. For example, a little celery balances a lot of cantaloupe (rockmelon). Check the locations of spinach, bananas, celery and cantaloupe on the detailed CaPNaK Chart.

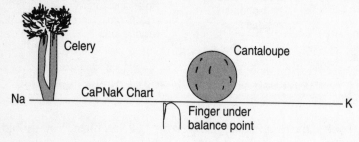

A little celery balances a lot of cantaloupe.

Health Effects

You can maintain the balance of your body-mind just like you have imagined balancing the chart. The foods on opposite sides of the balance point have complementary opposite effects on your body-mind. Now look at the following summary of these effects or symptoms.

Try to find some complementary opposite effects between the up and down directions, and also between the right and left directions. For example, feeling cold is a symptom in the left direction, feeling hot is a symptom in the right direction.* Celery is on the left side of the chart; if you eat enough celery you will feel cooler. Bananas are on the right side; if you eat enough bananas you will feel warmer.

You may be wondering why opposite directions on the chart have complementary effects. It is because the corresponding minerals have some complementary effects on the body-mind.

---

* Yang food makes heat move outward from the body; yin food makes heat move inward in the body. See Eating for Body Fluids Health.

Symptoms of overdose of calcium or underdose of phosphorus (alkalosis, from eating too much of the calcium-residue foods shown on the CaPNaK Chart)

Excessively calm, tranquil, lazy, careless
Put on fat easily
Large bones
Lack of muscle tone and strength
Sleepiness
Hypoactivity

Symptoms of overdose of sodium or under-dose of potassium (from eating too much of the sodium-residue foods shown on the CaPNaK Chart)

Excessively intense, irritable, angry, aggressive, short-tempered
Feel cold
Bags under the eyes
Excessive libido
Muscle tension and inflexibility
Excessive sweating, clamminess
Swelling of extremities
High blood pressure
Water retention
Backache

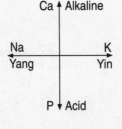

Symptoms of overdose of potassium or underdose of sodium (from eating too much of the potassium-residue foods shown on the CaPNaK Chart)

Excessively passive, timid
Feel hot
Feel faint
Feel drained
Sunken and dark around the eyes
Swollen lip, mouth ulcers
Headache
Short of breath
Low libido
Gas
Constipation, indigestion, abdominal bloating
Muscle weakness, shrinkage
Low blood pressure

Symptoms of overdose of phosphorus or underdose of calcium (acidosis from eating too much of the phosphorus-residue foods shown on the CaPNaK Chart)

Excessively anxious, paranoid, restless, worried
Hyperactivity
Lose fat easily
Thin bones
Muscle cramp
Insomnia
Acne
Scaly lips
Receding gums, bleeding gums loose teeth, tooth abscesses and decay
Cracked or broken bones
Osteoporosis
Arthritis

Symptoms of CaPNaK imbalance.

Helps you become more easy-going
Helps you relax and become tranquil
Helps thin people gain weight
Strengthens your bones and teeth
Stops muscle cramp
Reduces acne and scaly lips
Prevents or reduces receding or bleeding gums,
  loose teeth, tooth abscesses and decay
Prevents or reduces osteoporosis and arthritis
Helps you get to sleep easily
Helps you to slow down

Increases your drive and
  assertiveness
Cools you down
Removes dark patches
  under your eyes
Increases your sex drive
Increases your physical
  energy
Helps you sweat and
  build muscle
Stops or reduces
  dizziness, fainting, and
  shortness of breath
Lifts your blood pressure
Stops you feeling drained
Reduces swelling of lips
  and mouth ulcers
Helps stop many
  headaches
Reduces gas and
  constipation and helps
  digestion
Reduces abdominal
  bloating
Prepares you for hot
  weather

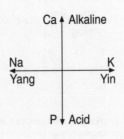

Reduces your
  agressiveness and
  intensity
Warms you up
Reduces sexual
  obsession
Loosens up your body
Reduces your blood
  pressure
Removes bags under
  your eyes
Prepares you for
  contemplative activity
Prepares you for cold
  weather

Speeds you up for peaks in activity
Arouses your concern and attention
Helps fat people to lose weight
Reduces your need for sleep
Improves muscle tone and strength

Positive effects of CaPNaK residues.

The Four Minerals

All foods contain four minerals in larger quantities than other minerals. These four primary minerals are the CaPNaK minerals: calcium (Ca), phosphorus (P), sodium (Na) and potassium (K).

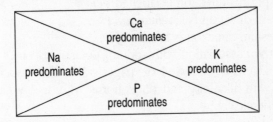

On the chart the background triangles indicate which mineral predominates in each food.

However, it is not as simple as positioning the foods on the chart according to their ratios of these minerals. A more useful method to set up the chart takes into account the physiological balance of these minerals in the body, and a more detailed explanation of the physiological basis of the CaPNaK Chart is given in Part 2. (It is not essential to read The CaPNaK Chart in Detail, pages 160–9, but it will give you a stronger basis for understanding this book.)

Understanding the CaPNaK Chart

Each of the vertical and horizontal axes shows a complementary pair of minerals. The distance from the central balance point shows the residual mineral left over from digestion of the food and, therefore, the strength of the effects on the body-mind. You will notice that the balance point on the chart is a little to the right of centre. That allows the chart to show the sodium-residue foods that are more extreme than the most extreme potassium-residue foods ('extreme' meaning far from the balance point).

Some of you will be familiar with food combining. CaPNaK balancing has nothing to do with food combining! Food combining relates to digestion of food, and is discussed in Eating for Digestion. CaPNaK balancing relates to the balance of your inner states, such as warm/cool, tense/relaxed, anxious/calm, etc.

Alkaline/Acid and Yin/Yang

Each of the four directions on the CaPNaK Chart is given another label besides the name of a mineral:

- the calcium direction is labelled *alkaline*
- the phosphorus direction is labelled *acid*
- the sodium direction is labelled *yang*
- the potassium direction is labelled *yin*.

The yang/yin association with sodium/potassium comes from macrobiotics, and is discussed on pages 47–8. The association of calcium with alkalinity and phosphorus with acidity can be explained chemically.*

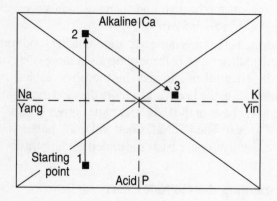

Tracing a path on the CaPNaK Chart of the state of the body-mind.

The labels yin, yang, acid or alkaline are sometimes used to indicate the set of body-mind symptoms (body-mind state) associated with a direction on the CaPNaK Chart. For example, in the miniature chart shown above, position 1 (the starting state) is an acid–yang

---

* The calcium ion in water tends to form an alkaline solution because it only weakly attracts bonding electrons in nearby water molecules, making it difficult for protons to be donated by the water. Conversely, the phosphate ion strongly attracts bonding electrons, resulting in acid solutions in water. Of course, there is ample water in the body-mind for these effects to emerge.

body-mind state—the body-mind state resulting from simultaneous excess phosphorus and sodium intake. Position 2 is an alkaline–yang state, and position 3 is a predominantly yin state.

Symptoms of Overdose

You can think of the effects of a residual mineral as symptoms of the body-mind overdosing with the residual mineral. The diagram on page 19 summarises some symptoms of imbalance in each of the four directions. Take another good look at the diagram now: it is the key to everyday use of the CaPNaK Chart.

Try to remember some of the symptoms in each direction so you can diagnose your body-mind state without referring to the diagram. At each moment you will be in a different CaPNaK state. Your body-mind state is steadily changing. By observing your state you can choose appropriate food to create the body-mind state you want at the time.

Some of the symptoms take years to appear. For example, arthritis may appear as acidity builds up in the body-mind. These symptoms may also take years to disappear even after the food intake is improved. Other symptoms (such as cooling or warming) appear or disappear in minutes or hours. These fast-changing symptoms can also be observed and controlled.

Note that many of these symptoms can also be seen as positive (see page 20). If the body-mind is suffering from the reverse symptom, and is then rebalanced, the effect is positive. For example, if the symptom is anxiety, then the symptom of laziness provided by a calcium-residual food source will often provide tranquillity. Thus, the CaPNaK Chart is not just a diagnostic tool, it is also a system of medicine where the food is the medicine, and the side effect is satiation!

Food Groups

Look at the CaPNaK Chart. You will notice that the foods cluster into groups. The following miniature CaPNaK Chart shows the locations of these food groups.

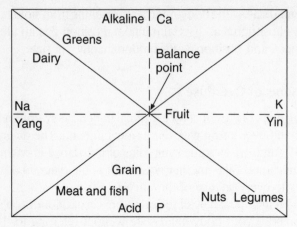

Overview map of food groups on the CaPNaK Chart.

The CaPNaK Chart includes many unhealthy foods such as meat, dairy products and grain, so even people who mostly prefer these foods can benefit from using the chart. However, where possible, the foods are shown according to their composition in a raw state without additives.

Sugar, oil and some other foods are at the balance point of the CaPNaK Chart. This is not because they are well-balanced sources of minerals, but because they are entirely mineral-deficient.

Is Fruit the Answer?

It is of great significance that the location of fruit near the central balance point makes it the most balanced food group for humans. This is further evidence that an eating system consisting mostly of fruit is a reasonable approach to nutrition.

An objection many people raise to fruitarianism is that fruit provides too much sugar (or fructose), thereby destabilising blood-sugar levels. In fact, this does not occur. Much of the sugar is bound into the cellular structure of the fruit. After the chewed particles enter the stomach, enzymes and stomach acid break the cell membranes at a controlled rate. Protein structures are dismantled in the stomach. This releases the sugar in a slow-release manner controlled by the body-mind.

Eventually this acid pulp (the chyme) is released to the duodenum. The slowly-releasing sugar then enters the bloodstream without provoking wild highs and lows of blood-sugar by insulin over-production. Actually, fruit is a hybrid carbohydrate—it contains both simple and complex carbohydrates.

Another positive factor with fruit, often overlooked, is that a fruit, as a living uncooked entity, contains an abundance of active enzymes. Some of these enzymes help in the digestion of the fruit. This frees the stomach, pancreas, and other digestive organs from some of their burden. The biochemical energy that the body-mind saves can be diverted to other important tasks, including boosting immunity. This is a partial explanation for the extraordinary resistance to infection and cancer displayed by live-food eaters.

The manufacturers of water filters may be disappointed to hear that fruit is a wonderful source of biologically purified water. In fact, there is so much water in fruit that fruitarians rarely need to drink anything. Eating a little more than 2 kg of fruit per day provides about 2 litres of water.

Fruit eating is also good news if you want to burn up some excess fat. In your cells fat burns in the flame of carbohydrate, and fruit is typically over 90 per cent carbohydrate. So your excess body fat is more easily burnt up when you eat more fruit.

Green-leaf Vegetables

It is very difficult or impossible to obtain adequate supplies of some minerals from fruit alone, the most important of these minerals being calcium. So it is advisable to eat green-leaf vegetables, which are an excellent source of minerals, including calcium. I recommend eating about 750 g raw greens per day. This will also provide an excellent source of protein. The essential amino acids in greens are a good complement to those in many fruits. (In *Diet for a Small Planet* (1975) Frances Moore Lappe stated that all eight essential amino acids should be eaten in every meal. This is erroneous, and she has since withdrawn that view.)

A quick look at the CaPNaK Chart reveals that most fruits are located on the potassium side of the central balance point. Thus, it is common to develop a need for sodium when eating mostly fruit. Many green-leaf vegetables are an excellent source of sodium, and are a useful addition to your diet for maintaining a vigorous sodium-potassium balance (i.e. other live foods are yin and put you in a passive state).

Suggested Daily Menu

The following daily menu is a good basis to build a Symbiotic menu around:

    4 sticks of celery (70 g per stick)
    500 g broccoli (one and a half heads)
    5 bananas (100 g per banana)
    6 large oranges (190 g per orange)
    20 g unhulled tahini (unhulled sesame seeds;
        pepitas can be added for zinc)

As you will only get about 4870 kilojoules from this, it would be wise to add more fruit. As it stands, it will provide you with following proportions:

	Kilojoules
Protein	18%
Fat	12% (polyunsaturated 48%, monounsaturated 38%, saturated 14%)
Carbohydrate	70%

Ratios like these are considered excellent by modern nutritionists (Pritikin & McGrady 1973).

Sceptics please note that this scanty, fruity menu provides 49 g protein, which is very close to the conventional recommended daily intake (RDI) for a 70 kg male!

I have checked the nutritional content of the sample day's menu using nutritional analysis software. The only nutrient that fell significantly short of the RDI was zinc; 72 per cent of the RDI was provided, so a 35 per cent increase in the quantities would meet all recommendations. I recommend that novice fruit-eaters eat approximately the suggested daily menu, and add to it a variety of fruit and vegetables. This way you can be sure you are getting complete, balanced nutrition, with the exception of vitamin B_{12} (see pages 61–3).

Animal Food and Cereals

For those wishing to supplement their diet with a little animal food, I made an analysis of the above menu with 30 g sardines added to ensure that the current RDI for vitamin B_{12} is met. The total kilojoules increased to 5166 kilojoules, with the following proportions:

	Kilojoules
Protein	19%
Fat	15% (polyunsaturated 44%, mono-unsaturated 37%, saturated 19%)
Carbohydrate	66%

It is very important for a fruit-eater to minimise the eating of cereals because of their digestive incompatibility with fruit, as mentioned earlier. If a cereal-based food is eaten, then no fruit should be eaten for an hour or so until the cereal has left the stomach. Grain is for the birds and beasts.

Millions of years of evolution have provided us with our own symbiotic foods that give us and our planet optimum health. An interesting example of symbiotic evolution of food is wheat. Wheat and the cereal grasses from which wheat was derived contain oestrogens (female sex hormones). This was the result of a symbiotic evolutionary mechanism for limiting the reproduction of those animal species eating these grasses (Pearson & Shaw 1982). Eaten in sufficient quantity, these oestrogens may adversely effect the testicles and sex drive in male humans.

The Symbiotic Groups

Within Symbiotics there are two main sub-groups: Fruitarians and Live Fooders.

Fruitarians

Mono-fruitarian (one kind of fruit at a time)
Frugivore (only fruit)
Herbo-fruitarian (fruit and green-leaf vegetables)
Herbo-pisco-fruitarian (raw fish as well)

Live-fooders

Bean-sproutarian (bean sprouts added to a fruitarian menu)
Grain-sproutarian (sprouted wheat bread added to a fruitarian menu; problems combining with fruit)
Grass-eater (wheat grass added to a fruitarian menu, usually medicinally).

Beware of being a Saprovore (eating decaying organic matter); eat your food as fresh as possible.

The transition to fruit-based eating behaviour is extremely difficult, because it requires extensive re-education of tastes, cravings, feeding patterns and cultural behaviour. The aspiring Symbiotic must uproot and reprogramme years of unconscious conditioning. Some people can do it instantly, others take decades to make the transition. However, for those pioneers who persist in exploring this symbiotic way of eating, the rewards are great.

The following chapters focus on how you can use the CaPNaK Chart in relation to particular aspects of your life. If you read the chapters in order you will better understand the information based on these preceding chapters. However, once you gain some familiarity with the use of the CaPNaK Chart, then random reference to any of the chapters should not create misunderstandings. For more detail on the Chart, see pages 160–9.

Eating for the Past

You have probably wondered what humans ate in the wild when they lived naturally like other animals. Fortunately, anthropologists have discovered a window through which they can investigate the eating habits of our early human ancestors. The quantity of tiny scratches, or microwear, on teeth enables an animal to be broadly classified as predominantly a carnivore, omnivore, herbivore or frugivore. The density of microwear reduces in that order, with frugivores showing almost no microwear.

A discovery by Dr A. Walker, reported in the *New York Times* in 1979, surprised anthropologists. He found that microwear on the teeth of fossils of hominids of the 12 million year period leading up to *Homo erectus* was that of frugivores. The microwear was indistinguishable from that of today's chimpanzees and orang-utans.

Homo erectus was the first form of human beings to migrate from Africa. This happened about a million years ago, and was made possible by their potential for omnivorous eating. They discovered tools and fire to process previously inedible foods such as hard cereals. However, human digestion has remained predominantly that of a frugivore, like the chimpanzee.

In her studies of primates, Katherine Milton (1993) found that those predominantly frugivorous also ate young green-leaf vegetables. In seasons when fruit became scarce they supplemented their eating with higher fibre foliage, which was lower in available energy. She found that chimpanzees and humans can digest fibre when necessary by fermenting the fibre in the gut. The transmission of food through the gut speeds up, so a larger amount of food is digested, maintaining the rate of energy input.

The wild chimpanzee eats 94 per cent fruit and leafy vegetables, and 6 per cent raw animal foods (including other monkeys)— hundreds of grams of fibre, compared with the 10 g eaten by the average modern human. Our commercially available fruit has more pulp and less fibre than wild fruit.

The evidence for the similarity between chimpanzee and hominid eating patterns and digestion suggests that we *Homo sapiens* are adapted for similar eating. Thus, eating predominantly fruit with a proportion of greens, and if necessary up to a maximum of 10 per cent raw animal foods (preferably less than 5 per cent), appears to be in harmony with our evolution. The proportion of greens should be increased during seasons of lower availability of fruit.

At best, hunting is a time-consuming and energetically expensive way of living. Chimpanzees do it as a last resort. When few trees are in fruit, chimpanzees fall back on high-fibre foods such as pith (spongy tissue in the stems and branches of plants). Only when high-fibre foods become scarce do they tend to hunt more frequently (Dunbar 1991). Unfortunately, this energy constraint on hunting must have diminished for humans when they developed tools and, eventually, weapons.

The rise of hunting finally led to depletion of wild animal stocks and the development of agriculture. The transition to cereal agriculture from the hunter-gatherer lifestyle occurred between 7000 and 10 000 years ago. A comparison of skeletal remains revealed that the agricultural populations were, on average, shorter (by about 10 cm), lighter (by about 7 kg) and more susceptible to skeletal diseases linked to their diet such as osteoporosis (Dunbar, 1991). They suffered chronic energy deficiency, and ate little meat or fruit.

Because of the reduced availability of fruit outside the tropical forests, *Homo erectus* found it necessary for survival to process and cook (mutilate) food. Civilised man found it necessary to grow and eat cereals. However, now we can cultivate orchards and vegetable gardens, and transport fruit and vegetables into regions where they cannot be grown. So at last it is becoming possible to return to our symbiotic foods and optimum health wherever we may live.

Eating for Evolution of Consciousness

Evolution involves gradual progression by natural selection of higher degrees of organisation of life. Your psychological consciousness, residing mainly in your nervous system, is part of your aliveness, and it, too, has the potential to become more highly organised. Deep organisation of consciousness brings clarity out of confusion, peace out of conflict, and satisfaction out of craving.

In any system, organisation is constructed from information and negentropy (the structural ordering of matter). Put another way, information brings harmony, and negentropy brings order to a system. Information and negentropy entering your nervous system are flows that help to organise your consciousness (Brook 1987). Information and negentropy entering your body-mind help to organise the consciousness of your body-mind.

For example, the information and negentropy you gain by eating an orange can contribute to your evolution of consciousness. The structure of fruit involves an enormous amount of negentropy that the tree has extracted from sunlight. The enzymes in fruit encode information on how to metabolise food by sequences of actions for breaking molecules. Food mutilated by heat loses negentropy and information, and the harmony and order in the molecular systems of the food is lost. Potentially, your evolution of consciousness is slowed, stopped, or reversed (in disease) by eating mutilated foods.

A tolerable post-modern definition of sin could be: 'Anything that stops evolution in consciousness is evil.' Sometimes you reach a point where you know through experience that some action, such as eating a certain food, is a barrier to your evolution of consciousness. Then it is time to replace that action with an action that promotes your growth.

Consciousness grows out of awareness. You can develop awareness of your eating patterns and their effects by keeping a food log. Here is an example.

Time	Food eaten	Notes
8 a.m.	Coffee	Sleepy
8.30 a.m.	Muesli and egg	Rushing
9.30 a.m.		Dead tired
10 a.m.	Pie and coke	Hungry
11 a.m.	Aspirin	Drained, headache
noon	Milkshake	
	Sausage sandwich	Belch! Stomach ache
[etc.]		

Record a food log for yourself over four or five days, and look for cause and effect connections between what you eat and the state of your body-mind. As your awareness develops, you will become interested in choices and directions. What shall I do—rob a bank or rob my liver? Or you may choose to reduce your risk of getting cancer.

'Food chakras' provide a map for exploring eating, and making choices. The transitions from one level to the next bring the body-mind into a more balanced, light and uncongested state. The following table shows the progression of food replacements.

As you move up the food chakras you bring the body-mind into a more alkaline state. This is because fewer phosphorus-residue and more calcium-residue foods are present. A temporary highly alkaline state, useful in promoting chakra development, can be induced through drinking certain vegetable juices (such as carrot and parsley juice) and by deep breathing.

People also attain this state in a highly aroused condition, such as when a traumatic situation occurs. In traumatic situations the breath becomes deep, and the pulse quickens. The body-mind hyperventilates, and carbon dioxide is removed from the bloodstream, which then becomes more alkaline. Instinctive brain responses for dealing with traumatic situations are aroused in association with this alkalinity, and the body-mind attains a transcendental state of awareness.

If you induce this temporary alkaline state, in non-traumatic circumstances using food and breathing, you can relive, integrate and release psychological traumas. This is the basis of breath-oriented therapies, widely used at present. With each release from the traumas of the past comes a new freedom in consciousness. Your capacity to sustain a transcendental alkaline state grows as you untie these psychophysical knots.

Similarly, you can use the CaPNaK Chart as a guide to the extremes of imbalance of your body-mind. For example, if you eat only potassium-residue foods for a day you will gain a deep

Food chakra	Stimulant	Sweetener	Minerals	Fat/Protein
7 Symbiotic	Juicy fruit	Sweet fruit	Green vegetables	Nuts
6 Vegan	Juice	Dried fruit	Cooked vegetables	Grains
5 Macrobiotic	Herbal tea	Honey	Miso	Beans
4 Vegetarian	Tea	Raw sugar	Vegetable salt	Dairy foods
3 Piscavore	Coffee	Sugar	Sea salt	Fish
2 Carnivore	Alcohol	Sweets	Sauce	Meat
1 Junkivore	Cigarettes	Drugs	Refined salt	Fat

understanding and sensitivity to the impact of different foods on the state of your body-mind.

Buddha told his disciples to eat what they are given, and not to tell people what to give them. In those days everyone knew they were vegetarians, but most Buddhists around the world now are non-vegetarian. Their attitude is that food is material, it is trivial, not spiritual. However, killing higher (sentient) life forms may harden the heart, and then spiritual growth in emotional sensitivity is delayed.

Of course, every second our immune system is killing bacteria and other parasites, and we squash insects whenever we walk outside. So to walk in peace it helps to recognise that life is a spectrum between higher and lower forms. The point is that where you draw the line, what killing you are willing to participate in, relates to your emotional sensitivity or depth of consciousness. It may be impossible for an enlightened person to eat meat. However, munching the odd grub in an apple will not harden the heart unless the brain has already softened.

Many people have enlightenment as their spiritual goal. Since enlightenment cannot be defined in dualistic terms, it may be more useful to consider my definition of enlivenment:

- can eat living food
- OK to feel all emotions
- OK to pursue goals
- enjoy sex
- the material world is significant
- time and space thought to exist
- body and health are considered important
- responsible for enjoying life with everyone
- may kill mosquitoes when attacked.

What is your spiritual aim? Do you fervently seek enlivenment? If you do, it is unwise to ignore entirely the traditional spiritual teachings. Meditation is a part of all major religions, but has been elaborated most thoroughly in Buddhist and Hindu teachings. Meditation has long been considered the key to the evolution of consciousness. There are three main forms of meditation: tantric (relation-centred), vipassana (observation-centred), and kundalini (action-centred).

Tantric meditation involves both observation and action in relation to others and the self. This includes inanimate others, such as a piece of fruit. You can treat eating as a tantric meditation just by being aware during the process.

Kundalini and vipassana styles can also apply to eating and digestion. For example, your second psychophysical chakra is located in your abdomen below your navel. If you contract your lower abdomen intentionally and with awareness, you are performing a kundalini meditation practice. This second chakra relates to desire for, and withdrawal from, sensation. Imbalance in this chakra can manifest physically, as in lower back pain. This back pain usually indicates an unstable orientation to withdrawal from sensation. An unstable orientation of desire for, and/or withdrawal from, food may appear as anorexia and/or bulimia, for example.

You can use meditative contraction of muscles associated with the second chakra to develop consciousness regarding sensation. For example, you can develop more conscious digestion.

Also, if you are a dedicated meditator, eating living food also reduces your digestive load, and eliminates some outer sources of distraction. Then you have more attention available for the inner journey.

Finally, here is a quote from Osho's *Rajneesh Bible* (vol. 3, Discourse 25, 23 January 1985):

> Devaraj has been of great help. He has dropped all milk products . . . from my food, and I feel really clean . . . For the first time in my life I am feeling at ease with food. In India it was impossible because everybody was harassing me: 'If you drop milk then there is nothing in the food' . . . Right now all of my difficulties have disappeared.

From this mystic's account, it is also possible to know your Self without knowing your health.

Eating for Bones and Soft Tissue Health

Plagues of termites are gnawing at our bones. We feed these termites with the grains that our health authorities recommend in ever-increasing portions. Do we wait until the roof collapses before we do anything? Not if we know about the termites. However, most of us don't know that the very frames of our bodies are dissolving. Nevertheless, the reasons for the damage are within our control.

Here is some physiological background. The body-mind releases parathyroid hormone, and retains calcitonin hormone, when there are low calcium levels or high phosphorus levels in the blood. This increases the amount of calcium removed from the bones (Guyton 1977). Foods such as grains and meats are high in phosphorus and low in calcium. When they are eaten excessively the body-mind removes calcium from the bones. This is simple but deadly serious! The plague is osteoporosis, and the termite is phosphorus.

Osteoporosis is a metabolic disorder usually defined as the loss of calcium from bone, and the loss of the supporting collagen framework on which the calcium is deposited. One out of four older women and one in seven older men suffer from this disabling and disfiguring condition. Nearly one woman in every thousand breaks a hip each year, and one in five of those dies within twelve months from complications (Goulder 1988). Although it may appear to be a disease of the elderly, in reality bone degeneration starts much earlier in life. Prevention of osteoporosis is a crucial consideration for men and women in their twenties and thirties.

Experiments on adult animals and humans indicate that the calcium requirement of adults consuming the typical high-phosphorus, high-protein, acidic Western diet is greater than on other more alkaline diets (Draper 1981). In addition, the consumption of calcium in industrialised countries is highly variable, depending largely on the consumption of dairy foods, usually the main source of calcium. Additional consumption of foods containing phosphate food additives could potentially overload the body-mind with phosphorus.

Low calcium or high phosphorus intake has a greater effect on the skeleton of younger adults than on that of aged adults. Also, bone loss is more severely increased by higher phosphorus intake than by lower calcium intake.

Animal experiments indicate that increased phosphate intake reduces excretion of calcium in the urine, but increases excretion in the faeces (Draper 1981). The question is: 'Are you flushing your bones down the toilet?' More skeletons are snaking their way down the sewers than we might have imagined!

In the laboratory, growing rats limit their phosphorus intake to about half the proportion eaten by adult rats. Higher intake of phosphorus depresses appetite and weight gain of adult rats and pigs. Significant decreases in bone mass have been observed in rodents fed on a diet with a Ca:P (calcium:phosphorus) ratio of 1:2 over the adult life span (Draper 1981). An American-style diet has the Ca:P ratio of about 1:1.6. Dairy products have a Ca:P ratio of about 1:0.75; However, they are high in phosphorus as well as calcium, so the reduced ratio is not so effective. Some people avoid dairy products without increasing their intake of green-leaf vegetables; they have a significantly worse ratio, and are most likely to suffer from osteoporosis.

Meat provides two major sources of acidity: phosphorus and sulphur-based proteins, which are more acidic than vegetable proteins. The consequent loss of calcium is demonstrated by the fact that female meat-eaters at age 65 have an average bone loss of 35 per cent, compared with 18 per cent for female vegetarians of the same age (EarthSave Foundation 1992).

On an average diet the body sheds about 300 mg calcium a day. The body absorbs about 35 per cent of the calcium in foods, so nutritional experts recommend that a minimum of 800–1000 mg calcium must be consumed daily to avoid the gradual dissolving of bone tissues. Babies' requirements are lower, and women's requirements are higher (up to 1500 mg per day if they are post-menopausal). Older people need more calcium because the ability to absorb calcium reduces with age (Goulder 1988).

Another factor in the calcium–phosphorus balance is that phosphorus can combine with calcium in the digestive tract. This, too, can prevent the absorption of calcium (Colbin 1986). It seems likely that people eating lower amounts of phosphorus have a lower requirement for calcium than the current recommendations. Until there are research results, I do not suggest a lower intake of calcium. However, I do suggest a lower consumption of phosphorus-residue foods. The CaPNaK Chart provides a clear indication of how to do this while increasing calcium-residue food intake.

Calcium has an alkaline effect in the blood, and phosphorus (as phosphate) has an acidic effect. So the calcium and phosphorus levels in the blood are related to the acid–alkaline balance. Hence, I have labelled the calcium–residue and phosphorus–residue directions on the CaPNaK Chart as alkaline and acid, respectively. Muscle tissue contains more phosphorus, and bone tissue contains more calcium. Think of the calcium–phosphorus axis as a bone-versus-muscle dimension.

A person who has built up calcium levels by eating large quantities of calcium-rich foods for many years (i.e. overdosed on calcium) is usually large-boned and fat. Conversely, the person who has built up phosphorus levels (i.e. overdosed on phosphorus) is usually thin-boned and underfat.

If you are one of the millions who often get muscle cramp, your condition is probably avoidable. You may just need to make some changes in what you eat to reduce your acidosis. Temporary reductions of acidity in the blood can temporarily improve some symptoms. However, most of these symptoms take a long time to improve permanently because the calcium level in the bones cannot be changed quickly. It takes years to recharge or discharge your body's calcium. Recharging your bones with calcium may be very difficult if you are older. Nevertheless, with appropriate nutrition you can at least halt depletion.

Summary of Overdose Symptoms

Symptoms of overdose of calcium or underdose of phosphorus (alkalosis from eating too much of the calcium-residue foods shown on the CaPNaK Chart)	Symptoms of overdose of phosphorus or underdose of calcium (acidosis from eating too much of the phosphorus-residue foods shown on the CaPNaK Chart)
Excessively calm, tranquil, lazy, careless	Excessively anxious, paranoid, restless, worried
Put on fat easily	Hyperactivity
Large bones	Lose fat easily
Lack of muscle tone and strength	Thin bones
Sleepiness	Muscle cramps
	Insomnia
	Acne
	Scaly lips
	Receding gums, bleeding gums, loose teeth, tooth abscesses, and tooth decay
	Cracked or broken bones
	Osteoporosis
	Arthritis

(Nutrition Search 1979)

Besides high phosphorus intake, there are two other important sources of calcium loss caused by foods. One is sodium, which pulls calcium with it out of the body when it is excreted. So, salt intake should be minimised to avoid calcium loss. The other is protein, which results in uric acid in the blood (Colbin 1986). This acidity is neutralised with calcium from the bones if it is present in excessive quantities. Look at the position of meat on the CaPNaK Chart. It is high in sodium- and phosphorus-residue, and is, of course, high in protein. That is a reason why meat is a potent contributor to calcium loss.

High protein (meat) intake has been shown to increase calcium excretion in the urine and removal from the bones. Evidence published in the *Journal of American Geriatrics* (Barzel 1982) showed that meat and other high-protein foods, and most grains

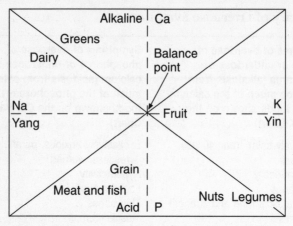

The CaPNaK Chart, showing the location of food groups.

and starches increase calcium excretion and bone loss. In particular, the new lower-fat animal foods currently being promoted are a potential source of excessive protein.

Inuit (Eskimos) traditionally obtained calcium from the bones of marine and land mammals and the soft bones of fish. Although the hunting tradition is still strong, bone chewing is rarely practised now. Consequently, their calcium intake is low and the calcium to phosphorus ratio is wide. Inuit have a rate of bone loss 15–20 per cent higher than other North Americans (Draper & Scythes 1981).

African women consume 350–500 mg calcium daily, but do not lose calcium in their urine. This is partly because they eat mainly corn and vegetables, a far lower protein intake (Robbins 1987).

The protein myth that stipulates that consumption of large amounts of protein is beneficial is probably the most pervasive 'Big Lie' about food. Studies of other cultures show that one part protein to seven parts carbohydrate is best (by weight or kilojoules): this is the proportion consumed by the Hunzas (in the Himalayas) and Vilacabambans (in Ecuador), the longest-lived people on Earth besides the Symbiotics (Colbin 1986). Symbiotics get this proportion of complete protein by eating about 750 g greens every day.

You may notice on the CaPNaK Chart that white bread is much less acid than wholemeal bread. This is mainly because the white bread shown has milk powder in its ingredients. However, don't go rushing back to white bread for the calcium. Milk powder and other dairy products have big problems.

Two problems with human consumption of dairy foods are the high protein and phosphorus contents of dairy foods. This works well for calves, which grow much faster than humans. In humans the protein contributes additional acidity, which is not shown by the calcium–phosphorus balance. Again, the phosphorus can combine with calcium in the digestive tract and prevent the absorption of calcium.

A third and important problem is that dairy products stimulate the excretion of mucus in the digestive tract. This is more easily noticed in the nose and throat when you eat dairy products after a long period of avoidance. Mucus is excreted to protect the mucous membrane. However, when it is repeatedly excreted it becomes a breeding ground for infection and a blockage to nutrient absorption. The factors in dairy products that stimulate the production of mucus seem to be related to the fatty components. Low-fat dairy products are not so mucogenic.

The vast majority of humans do not retain the ability to digest the lactose in milk after infancy. Those who can digest lactose escape the reactions, which include cramps, bloating, intestinal gas and diarrhoea.

Fruitarians, live fooders and vegans can ensure they are getting enough calcium by eating at least 750 g green-leaf vegetables every day. Pregnant, lactating and post-menopausal women, and men over 60, need more calcium (Goulder 1988). They should eat 1–1½ kg green-leaf vegetables every day if they don't eat dairy products. Fruit alone does not supply sufficient amounts of calcium.

To illustrate this I have calculated for each fruit the quantity needed to provide a requirement of 1000 mg calcium a day:

18 oranges (3.3 kg)
or 83 apples (15 kg)
or 167 apricots (6.3 kg)

or 18 cantaloupes (7.1 kg)
or 56 figs (2.8 kg)
or 83 bananas (12.5 kg)
or 6.4 kg grapes
or 43 mangoes (13 kg)
or 6 kg pineapples
or 14 kg watermelon.

Oranges and figs are the only fruits that come close to being an adequate source. Oranges should be a staple food for herbo-fruitarians, but orange juice without the pulp is not a good source of calcium. You can see on the CaPNaK Chart that orange juice is high in phosphorus and low in calcium, and is therefore acidic. Whole oranges are alkaline.

Spinach, beet greens, Swiss chard (silverbeet) and parsley contain significant amounts of oxalic acid, and should be eaten only in small quantities (note that cooking destroys oxalic acid). Oxalic acid interferes with the availability of calcium and magnesium from these greens. Broccoli is one of the best sources of calcium for your food-dollar. Collards and sum choy are also highly recommended. See the CaPNaK Chart for high-calcium-residue greens.

Use a blender to liquefy your greens, but preferably not a juice extractor because then you don't get the whole food unless you stir it back in—there is usually a lot of calcium in the pulp.

Nightshades (including potatoes, tomatoes, eggplant, and all kinds of peppers) are high in alkaloids. These are not recom-mended, since they interfere with the calcium and phosphate in the blood and bones, and may contribute to the calcification of organs and joints.

If you cannot consume 750 g greens daily, then, besides citrus fruit, find some other good source of calcium. Some alternatives are: unhulled sesame seeds; unhulled tahini (sesame paste, not hulled tahini or hulled sesame seeds, which are stripped of the husks containing calcium; unfortunately, the husks also contain phytic acid which reduces the total calcium absorbed); tofu (not nigari tofu, which is low in calcium); low-salt cheese; low-fat yogurt; or calcium tablets. Safer is better than sorrier. Check the location of these foods on the CaPNaK Chart.

If you have diagnosed bone problems and need to take a calcium supplement, take one with about 1 part magnesium to 2 parts calcium (Nutrition Search 1979). Your body-mind needs calcium with magnesium (300 mg/day of magnesium, and 5 mg/day of manganese) to form hard–tooth enamel and to avoid calcium accumulation in the kidneys. Note that bone-based calcium tablets (calcium hydroxyl apatite) may not contain sufficient magnesium, etc. The calcium to magnesium ratio in broccoli is 1.4:1, and in unhulled sesame seeds 1:1, so they provide more than sufficient magnesium (based on data extracted from the nutritional analysis data base). Calcium citrate is one of the most completely absorbed form of calcium (Goulder 1988). If you (or a blood relative) have had a kidney stone, you should not increase your calcium intake without the approval of your physician.

Essential fatty acids help the body absorb calcium and deposit it in bone. Essential fatty acids are special acids that cannot be manufactured by the body, and are only required in small quantities from foods. Nuts, seeds and avocado are good sources of these acids.

If you are a woman, do not wait until menopause before you become concerned about your bone health. Bone health is determined well before menopause. However, menopausal women can still prevent further bone loss, particularly with load-bearing exercise. Walking is one of the best load-bearing exercises because your weight is supported by your entire skeleton. With swimming much of your body weight is carried by the water; and on a bicycle the seat carries part of your weight.

A good way to get feedback about the influence of your current diet on your acid–alkaline state is to test the acid–alkaline balance of your urine. Buy some blue litmus paper from a pharmacy, and swipe some through your midstream urine. If the litmus paper turns red or pink it is likely that you have been eating too much acidic food; if it stays blue or violet then you are probably eating more alkaline food. The litmus test indicates the current trend of your acid–alkaline balance, rather than the long-term acid–alkaline state of your body-mind. While you are adjusting your eating habits do the litmus test every day for feedback.

If you have diagnosed calcium deposits in your kidneys or

around your joints causing pain, it may not be that you are eating too much calcium-residue food, you may be eating too much acidic phosphorus-residue food. Calcium removed from the bones to balance acidity may not be properly excreted, and may be deposited in tissue.

You can have too much of a good thing, and calcium is no exception. Increased alkalinity of urine increases the risk of renal calcium-stone formation. Doctors recommend 2–3 litres of urine output each day for people with renal calcium stones (Kincaid-Smith 1993). If you are eating 90 per cent of your food raw, then it is likely that your daily urine output is at least 2 litres. This reduces your risk of renal stone formation.

Eating for Body Fluids Health

Every day millions of us wind up feeling drained. Sometimes we feel hot, dizzy, short of breath, or get a headache. At other times we feel cold, or intense and irritable, or aggressive. The good news is that these are symptoms that we can control. With the aid of the CaPNaK Chart you can gain this control just by becoming more aware of the effects on your body-mind of what you eat.

When you eat more sodium-residue foods the extracellular fluid (fluid outside the body's cells, page 165), including the blood volume, tends to increase. Changes in blood volume are always small, but blood volume varies in proportion to extracellular fluid volume (Guyton 1977). Blood pressure also tends to increase, the nerves fire more intensely, and muscle contraction becomes stronger. When you start to feel drained and weak, try a large salad or carrot and celery juice. Otherwise, simply chew two or three sticks of celery or a roll of green leaves to boost your sodium level.

Twenty minutes later you may find it hard to believe that you were feeling drained, but don't take it to the other extreme. Too much sodium over-excites the kidney–adrenal system, which may put you in a hostile frame of mind.

A friend used the CaPNaK Chart for a couple of years to rebuild his alkalinity, while ignoring the sodium–potassium aspect. One day he told me he had finally discovered the benefits of the sodium–potassium dimension. He had tried celery as a stimulant: now he swears it is as strong as coffee.

Choose your high sodium-residue foods from the left side of the CaPNaK Chart. It is a good idea to get your calcium when you are eating high-sodium foods; of course, living green leaves are the best choice. Make a sandwich of leaves, preferably without bread.

When you eat more potassium-residue foods, the extracellular fluid volume decreases. Also, blood pressure decreases, blood vessels near the skin contract, and muscle tension reduces. You can become aware of these effects after about 20 minutes. So, if you are feeling physically cold or hostile, eat a banana or an avocado to boost your potassium level. Bananas are nature's convenience food, with superb packaging. However, beware: they are loaded with potassium, and eating just two or three at one time can throw out your fluid balance.

Choose your high potassium-residue foods from the right side of the CaPNaK Chart. Most fruits are on the potassium-residue side of the balance point. They are a better choice than nuts, grains and potato, which are also strongly acidic.

The following lists of symptoms will help you keep track of your condition.

Symptoms of overdose of potassium or underdose of sodium (from eating too much of the potassium-residue foods shown on the CaPNaK Chart)

Excessively passive, timid
Feel hot
Feel faint
Feel drained
Sunken and dark areas around the eyes
Swollen lips, mouth ulcers
Headache
Shortness of breath
Low libido
Gas
Constipation, indigestion, abdominal bloating
Muscle weakness
Muscle shrinkage
Low blood pressure

Symptoms of overdose of sodium or underdose of potassium (from eating too much of the sodium-residue foods shown on the CaPNaK Chart)

Excessively intense, irritable, angry, aggressive, short-tempered
Feel cold
Bags under the eyes
Excessive libido
Muscle tension and inflexibility
Excessive sweating, clamminess
Swelling of extremities
High blood pressure
Water retention
Backache

(Nutrition Search 1979)

You can change most of these symptoms in a matter of minutes by eating 100–200 g of one of the counteracting foods shown on the opposing side of the CaPNaK Chart. Monitoring your sodium–potassium balance must become a continuous process if you wish to maintain peak performance of your body-mind. An obvious indication is under your eyes. If you have an excess of extracellular fluid, the bags under your eyes fill with fluid and swell out. This is a yang symptom, which can be rebalanced by a yin food such as banana (eat two). If you lack extracellular fluid, the bags shrink down and the dark vascular tissue underneath shows through as dark patches. This is a yin symptom, which can be rebalanced by a yang food such as celery (eat three sticks).

You can use the CaPNaK Chart to work out what will happen if you eat salted French fries! It really depends how much salt is on them. If you are lucky there may be just enough salt to balance the excess potassium of the potato.

Finally, a word about Macrobiotics. Many people are becoming familiar with the yin and yang classification, and what it means for the conditions of the body-mind. Sagen Ishizuka, the Japanese doctor who developed the original macrobiotic method, based it on the sodium–potassium balance. Accordingly, on the CaPNaK Chart I have labelled the sodium-residue direction 'yang' and the potassium-residue direction 'yin'.

Considerable contradictions arise when food is categorised using the one-dimensional yin–yang system. A well-known macrobiotic author, Herman Aihara (1982), strongly supports the view that the two dimensions of yin–yang and acid–alkaline are necessary to reduce the ambiguities. Also, in contrast to modern Macrobiotics, I have based the CaPNaK Chart solely on nutritional data so the positioning of the foods does not depend on subjective judgements.

When George Ohsawa defined yin and yang in Macrobiotics he intentionally switched their traditional association with contraction and expansion as follows:

Yang: heat. Traditionally: expansive. Macrobiotic: contractive.
Yin: cool. Traditionally: contractive. Macrobiotic: expansive.

To remove the confusion created by Ohsawa, I propose the following definition, which restores the scientific association of contraction with coolness and expansion with heat.

Yang: warmth and expansion outside, coolness and contraction inside
Yin: coolness and contraction outside, warmth and expansion inside.

This definition removes the contradiction of a yang salty food improving muscle contraction (inside), while also expanding blood volume near the skin (outside).

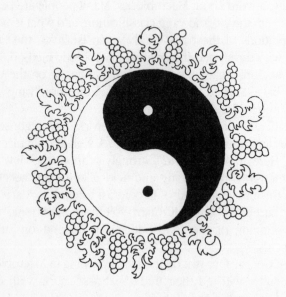

Eating for Energy

Fruit is racing fuel for humans, as well as for many other primates. Vegetables are about half the energy density of fruit, but they are a good source of vitamin B, and electrolytes such as sodium. Nature's power-boosting additives help the racing fuel reach the cells of the body-mind where it is needed. Grains are higher in kilojoules, but their complex carbohydrate kilojoules are less accessible because they have to be broken down. In addition, many grains barely contain enough vitamin B to cover their own breakdown. This may be one reason why many grain-eaters feel the need to take multi-vitamin pills. Proteins and fats are even more sluggish sources of energy because they are slow to digest.

On some occasions you may need energy that will last many hours. You have a choice: eat high-energy-density foods containing complex carbohydrates, fats, and proteins; or load up on fruit. I mean really load up, so that the whole intestine is full of fruit (and some greens, naturally)! This 'intestinal loading' with fruit is a basic principle for a high-energy symbiotic lifestyle. Erase any belief that a single stomachful of fruit can keep you going all day. You would be burning body fat (or is that body-mind fat?), which you may need for winter insulation.

A typical day's symbiotic eating pattern is given on the next page. Adjustments can be made for other climates and seasons; refer to later chapters.

This eating pattern of about fifteen average-sized pieces of fruit (about 100 g) would provide enough kilojules for a warm spring or autumn day when you are not very active. You should aim to eat at least five pieces of fruit before 10 a.m. to get an energetic high blood-sugar level start for the day. The nuts should include pump-

49

Time	Food	Comments
8 a.m.	2 bananas	A good warm-up food.
9 a.m.	1 orange, 150 g broccoli	A good start for calcium.
9.30 a.m.	2 kiwi fruit, 1 avocado	A kilojoule booster.
10 a.m.	1 peach, 100 g green-leaf vegetables	Sodium for activity.
11 a.m.	2 plums, 100 g grapes	More energy juice.
12 noon	1 rockmelon	Fluid for sweat.
1 p.m.	300 g green-leaf vegetables	A mineral feast.
1.30 p.m.	25 g nuts	More proteins and fats.
2 p.m.	1 orange	Peel yourself a drink.
3 p.m.	1 kiwi fruit, 200 g grapes	More racing fuel.
5 p.m.	2 bananas, 100 g green-leaf vegetables	Potassium for warmth.
6 p.m.	¼ avocado, 100 g broccoli	More calcium.
7 p.m.	1 orange	Eat a drink.

kin seeds for extra zinc, and unhulled sesame seeds for extra calcium, though the 750 g greens will ensure an adequate calcium intake.

We must distinguish between eating for mental or physical energy. The brain burns only carbohydrate for energy, but the muscles burn both carbohydrate and fat. So, the more physical work you do, the more fat you should eat: if you are digging ditches you might eat as much as two avocados a day. Avocados contain about 80 per cent fat. However, beware of the very significant health risks of excessive fat intake. This applies particularly to free fats and oils, which have been extracted from foods. (See Eating for Longevity for more information about fats.)

It is advisable to eat the minimum total food you can, without undesirable weight loss. Besides the health and financial benefits, eating less results in sleeping less and living more.

Eating for Digestion

Indigestion can be a pain in the gut, or it can be simply enervating. Who needs it! Buy yourself some pills and ignore the consequences? No, there is a better way. You may just need to apply a little knowledge about the what, how, and when of eating and digestion.

Anybody wishing to explore this crucial question more fully would do well to read *Fit for Life*, a bestseller by Harvey and Marilyn Diamond.

The Diamonds recommend that the bulk of food should be eaten within a period of about eight hours each day. The body-mind is then given adequate time for the processes of assimilation and elimination:

9 a.m. to 5 p.m.	Appropriation (eating and digestion)
5 p.m. to 1 a.m.	Assimilation (absorption and use)
1 a.m. to 9 a.m.	Elimination (waste collection and disposal)

The times shown above are not the same as in *Fit for Life*: the Diamonds recommended that appropriation should start at noon, but this is not good advice since it is established fact that you should eat well in the morning to avoid problems with low blood-sugar levels. According to traditional Chinese medicine the stomach and spleen are energised during appropriation; the kidneys during assimilation; and the liver and gall bladder during elimination.

All three body cycles function most easily when supplied with the enzyme-rich juices from fruits and vegetables. Fruit requires less energy for its digestion than any other whole food.

According to *Fit for Life*, any food that is not a fruit or a vegetable is 'concentrated' and requires special treatment by the stomach. The human body-mind is not equipped to digest more than one 'concentrated' food in the stomach at a time. This observation is the basis of the following principles of food combining. Nothing streamlines the appropriation cycle more than adhering to the principles of food combining. Improperly combined food rots in the stomach, and cannot be assimilated.

The main principles of food combining, summarised from *Fit for Life*, are:

- *Most important:* Fruit should never be eaten with or immediately following anything. Eat it on an empty stomach.
- In one meal, combine no more than one 'concentrated' food with vegetables.
- After eating other food, wait for the following times before eating fruit again:

> Salad or raw vegetables—2 hours
> Meal without flesh (meat, fish or poultry)—3 hours
> Meal with flesh—4 hours
> Any improperly combined meal—8 hours.

- Do not overeat, and do not undereat! Do be satisfied!

I agree with these principles of food combining, but I think that to avoid combining greens with fruit is unnecessary and unnatural. I do not notice any problem when I combine raw green-leaf vegetables with fruit (except for melons). Howler monkeys think so too: 'Having found a preferred food, they did not sate themselves. Instead they seemed driven to obtain a mixture of leaves and fruits, drawn from many plant species'; those species of monkey with a larger brain tended to eat more fruit and less leaves (e.g. lighter brain, 42 per cent fruit; heavier brain, 72 per cent fruit) (Milton 1993).

You may be wondering why this grazing is so important. By 'grazing' I mean eating whenever you are hungry. Preferably have many snacks instead of a few big meals, but allow time between grazing sessions.

You may ask: 'Isn't the stomach just an acid bath?' This brings us back to enzymes, and a deeper discussion of the advantages of raw, unheated foods.

Enzymes are involved in every process inside your body-mind. Each enzyme has a particular function, such as digesting carbohydrates or proteins or fats, or building tissue. As you grow older, your body-mind gradually loses the capacity to make enzymes, and consequently your internal processes slow down. Eventually, a shortage of enzymes results in serious health problems.

Your enzymes can be preserved and replenished by eating live food, which contains an abundance of enzymes. Food enzymes are destroyed by heat during food mutilation (cooking). Long heating at 48°C, or short heating at 65°C, destroys all enzymes. Every time you turn on your stove or oven, you create enzyme-deficient food, which imbalances your organs and leads to disease. Your white blood cell count increases after eating heated food, indicating that your body-mind is on the defensive. This does not occur after eating living food (Santillo 1987).

People who eat cereal (rice) with almost every meal develop an enlarged pancreas. This indicates a high demand for pancreatic enzymes, and thus too much stress on the pancreas. Also, older people have far less digestive enzymes available, so more undigested foods rot in their intestines. Chronically diseased people also have less enzymes in their body fluids. As their disease worsens their enzyme levels decrease (Santillo 1987).

Instead of forcing the body-mind (and pancreas) to do all the work, symbiotic evolution has created enzymes in food to aid digestion. A fraction of food enzymes can be absorbed in the intestines and used in other internal processes besides digestion (Santillo 1987).

Not all enzymes are destroyed in your stomach; many are merely inactivated by your stomach acidity and then reactivated in your intestines. However, this inactivation of enzymes does not occur in the upper part of your stomach—the enzyme stomach. Food remains in your enzyme stomach, where no acid secretion or peristalsis takes place, for 30–60 minutes after eating. In your enzyme stomach the enzymes in living food and your saliva predigest the food.

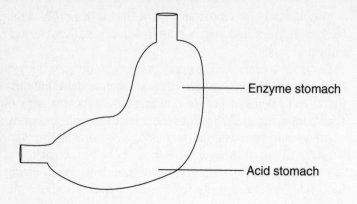

Enzyme stomach

Acid stomach

If you eat living food, your body-mind is relieved of the burden of producing large amounts of digestive enzymes later, when the food leaves your stomach. After predigestion of food in the enzyme stomach, the lower part of your stomach secretes acid and enzymes, and continues the digestive process, but less stomach acid is secreted if living food is eaten. The food enzymes from the enzyme stomach are then even more effective in the less acidic environment.

The following flow diagram summarises the important effects of enzyme-rich foods in the body-mind.

Food enzymes
- *Unabsorbed*, help digestion

  ↓

  reduce semi-digested substances entering the bloodstream

  ↓

  reduce consumption of internal enzymes

- *Absorbed*, help in other internal processes

  ↓

  reduce consumption of internal enzymes

The following flow diagram shows important effects of eating enzyme-depleted food.

Heated enzyme-depleted food
- *Slower digestion* (especially older people)
  ↓
  partially fermenting and rotting food in intestines
  ↓
  toxins and gas
  ↓
  degeneration and disease.

- *Higher demand for internal enzymes*
  ↓
  enlargement of enzyme-secreting glands
  ↓
  imbalance and exhaustion of endocrine system
  ↓
  stress and disease.

- *Depletion of internal enzymes*
  ↓
  body-mind energy loss
  ↓
  semi-digested substances enter bloodstream
  ↓
  leukocytosis: increased white blood cell count
  ↓
  immune system over-worked
  ↓
  other internal processes deteriorate
  ↓
  ageing and disease

When you are just starting to eat a lot of fruit, view any temporary discomfort as a body-mind cleansing process taking place and health beginning to return. Fewer than 10 per cent of people experience any discomfort. A friend quickly noticed he had worms —and the worms were not at all pleased with their new fruit diet!

Fit for Life gives a guide to the priority order of foods eaten over a day:

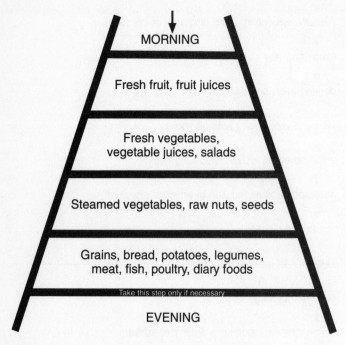

↓

MORNING

Fresh fruit, fruit juices

Fresh vegetables, vegetable juices, salads

Steamed vegetables, raw nuts, seeds

Grains, bread, potatoes, legumes, meat, fish, poultry, diary foods

Take this step only if necessary

EVENING

Climb down the Energy Ladder.

When you want to combine several foods together, use the food-combining chart on the opposite page. Foods sharing a common border can be digested together, and may be combined in one eating. Foods not sharing a common border cannot be digested simultaneously, and should not be combined in one eating.

Food-combining examples: acid fruits, greens and avocado all share borders, and may be eaten together. Dairy foods and subacid fruits do not share a border, and may not be eaten together. You may combine cheese with a vegetable salad; or citrus fruit with a vegetable salad; but do not combine cheese, vegetable salad, and

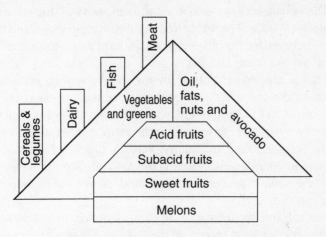

Sapoty's Snack Shack food-combining chart.

citrus fruit together, because dairy and acid fruit do not share a border and combine badly. Similarly melons and subacid fruit combine badly. Protein foods such as legumes and fish combine badly with each other, and are shown separated from each other in different chimneys; they combine well only with vegetables.

Here are some of the foods in these groups:

- **Acid fruit:** blackberry, grapefruit, kumquat, lemon, lime, orange, pineapple, plum, pomegranate, raspberry, strawberry, tangerine. (Note that many of these fruits are only superficially acidic. When the fruit is digested, the result may be acid or alkaline as indicated by the position on the CaPNaK Chart.)
- **Sub-acid fruit:** apple, apricot, blueberry, cherry, fig, grape, kiwi fruit, mango, nectarine, papaya (paw paw), peach, pear.
- **Sweet fruit:** banana, date, dried fruit, persimmon, raisin.
- **Melons:** cantaloupe, honeydew melon, watermelon.
- **Vegetables:** artichoke, asparagus, beetroot, broccoli, capsicum, carrot, celery, cucumber, green bean, leafy greens, parsnip, pea, radish, summer squash (zucchini), sweet corn, turnip.
- Potatoes are included among cereals and legumes.

Now, assuming that you are food-combining correctly, you can still have problems with digestion that can be explained with the

CaPNaK Chart. Let's say you eat some dates and two bananas. A few hours later you will probably find yourself feeling weak, and with your abdomen feeling bloated. You may have loose stools, concentrated yellow urine, and gas.

What is happening? Your body-mind has absorbed potassium-residue from the dates and bananas (see their position on the CaPNaK Chart). Consequently, your intestines are not contracting properly nor absorbing water into the extracellular fluids, so your stools become loose and watery. Partially digested food starts to ferment in your bowels, resulting in gas. Your body-mind tries to conserve sodium and extracellular fluid, so your urine becomes concentrated.

You can quickly rebalance all this discomfort by eating some sodium-residue food shown on the CaPNaK Chart, a few hundred grams of leafy greens for example. In less than an hour you will notice your strength has returned, and your abdomen contracting! If you have meditative, yogic or similar experience, you can help the digestive process. Direct your attention to your abdomen by stretching or contracting related muscles.

Gas or flatulence is so universal that it is considered natural. Anyone who has lived on properly combined living food without grain knows this is not so. It is not natural or healthy to have excessive gas; it is a sign of the presence of toxic fermentation in the bowels due to bad food combining. This fermentation produces toxic and acidic chemicals that are destructive and unbalancing to the body-mind.

When you combine a little grain with fruit, large amounts of fructose are present in the intestine in combination with incompletely digested carbohydrates. Your intestine moves the fructose-rich mixture through too quickly for proper absorption. Then unabsorbed fermentable types of carbohydrate from the grain result in bacterial action, forming gases. A small amount of fruit can be eaten after a grain meal without serious indigestion because the fructose-deficient mixture moves more slowly, allowing absorption to occur.

You will also cause gas and bloating if you do not chew your food enough. Saliva contains ptyalin (an amylase), which helps digest carbohydrates. When the food reaches the duodenum the carbohydrate digestion is completed by pancreatic enzymes. If your food has not been chewed enough, then the pancreatic enzymes cannot cope with the amount of undigested carbohydrate. The carbohydrates then ferment. So remember to chew your food so much that you drink it, rather than swallow it.

A related cause of flatulence is intestinal irritation by certain foods, such as chillies and unripe bananas. Many gases formed during digestion are usually absorbed, but when irritation occurs some are expelled before absorption.

When you eat foods that are distant from the central balance point, your digestion can be thrown off balance. This is because the full impact of what you have eaten is experienced by your body-mind after some delay. This can amount to ten or more hours for meats or grains. If you also delay your rebalancing efforts, then your body-mind state can bounce around the CaPNaK Chart for days! You may find this exciting, but more likely it will cause a disruption.

If you need some antacid, try substituting high calcium-residue foods, such as broccoli (see the CaPNaK Chart), for pills. The alkalinity of the calcium neutralises the acidity of high protein and high phosphorus-residue foods.

Finally, here are two points for would-be Symbiotics.

- I recommend grazing as a style of eating, with awareness of completion of digestion in your stomach before refilling it. This means not eating for at least half an hour, preferably one hour, after grazing on fruit and leafy greens. When you eat fruit, eat enough to fill your stomach comfortably (two or three pieces).
- Drinking water (and herb teas) can dilute digestive juices and nutrients. It is usually unnecessary to drink because unmutilated (uncooked) fruit and vegetables contain buckets of water. Try eating fruit to quench your thirst—fruit is more nutritious than water! People seem to think I am an alien when I tell them I do not routinely drink water! However, you may need to drink as well if you are very active in hot weather.

Eating for Vitamins and Minerals

Government surveys in developed countries show that many people lack sufficient vitamin A and C; the B vitamins (thiamine, pyridoxine and riboflavin), as well as calcium, iron and magnesium—60 per cent of the people with deficiencies show no overt signs (Berger 1985).

Common indications of vitamin deficiency are:

- frequent colds and flu
- ear, eye, nose or throat infections
- low energy
- swollen glands
- digestive problems
- blood disorders
- nervousness
- sleep problems
- irritability
- poor concentration
- anxiety
- weight problems.

Vitamins are the most important building block for immunity; especially vitamin C. The more vitamin C you eat, the greater is the weight of tissues in your immune system such as the thymus and lymph nodes, and the better they work to fight germs; if you eat mainly fresh fruit, you will automatically get sufficient quantities.

The meat industry is presently running a media campaign promoting meat as a better source of iron than vegetables. It is true that iron from animal foods is absorbed better than iron from green-leaf vegetables eaten alone. However, the vitamin C from many fruits (especially citrus) and vegetables help transform iron from the fruit and vegetables into the more readily absorbed form. So, eat vitamin

C-rich foods at the same time as iron-rich greens if you want to minimise your meat intake. Green-leaf vegetables, broccoli, beans and peas are rich in iron, and broccoli also has plenty of vitamin C.

Women need 18 mg iron each day. Green-leaf vegetables provide about 3 mg per 100 g, so you will meet the best part of your iron needs by eating over half a kilo of greens every day (Nutrition Search 1979). However, oxalic acid in certain greens (for example, beet greens, chives, parsley and spinach) reduces iron absorption by binding iron. Women should eat peas regularly to ensure their iron intake is sufficient; an extra 200 g raw peas a day would give a good boost to the usual intake of greens.

There is conflicting evidence about the nutritional benefits of organically grown food. Some studies have shown significantly higher vitamin and mineral levels, and others have not. Even if it is found that there is no nutritional advantage over conventionally grown produce, the other advantages of organically grown produce are great. Organic farming creates healthy plants and soil. The soil is improved instead of being denatured and eroded. Organically grown food does not contribute non-food chemicals to your body-mind. Organic farmers and distributors deserve financial support from your food dollars.

Pesticide residue in non-organically grown fruit and vegetables creates an increased need for vitamin B_6: bananas are a good source of B_6 from fruit. Two bananas a day will provide your daily requirement of about 1.5 mg B_6.

Some fruitarians believe that tropical fruit provides sufficient quantities of all nutrients. Contrary to this brave belief, I do not think fruit alone is adequate for long-term health, particularly regarding calcium and B_{12}.

I have already discussed calcium at length. I reiterate that eating 750 g green-leaf vegetables each day, in addition to 1 or 2 kg fruit, provides adequate calcium to prevent bone loss. This quantity of greens will also provide enough amino acids (protein), B vitamins (except B_{12}, perhaps), and other vitamins and trace minerals. Add a few nuts and seeds (20–30 g) or avocado (70 g) as a source of fats, etc., and optimum health will eventually be your reward—until your body runs low on its stores of B_{12}.

I once read about a doctor who went to India to study why the vegans there do not suffer from B_{12} deficiency. He checked out their diet, and could not find any source of B_{12}. Eventually, in frustration, he decided to take an Indian back to England and keep him eating exactly the same diet there. In England the Indian soon developed a B_{12} deficiency. Eventually the doctor found that it was the weevils and other tiny insects and bacteria in Indian foods that provided the B_{12}! This could become a big problem in India as they 'improve' their food storage and processing systems.

If you only eat vegetable foods that have had the insects sprayed out of them, then you may eventually begin to suffer from symptoms of B_{12} deficiency. This may take five to fifteen years. Anaemia, numbness, or memory loss are some symptoms to watch for. Brain damage similar to alcoholism can result from long-term deficiency of B_{12}. It is wise to get your B_{12} level checked by a doctor every year or so if you are in the vegan risk-group.

Even such dedicated vegetarians as grazing animals like cows get B_{12} from insects and soil bacteria in the grass they eat. This is irrespective of any internal synthesis a cow may have.

Tempeh (fermented soybeans) and some seaweeds, to my knowledge, are the only vegetable foods that provide B_{12} in adequate quantities to meet the recommended dietary intake of 3 mcg. However, you would have to eat about 100 g a day.

In 1987 a joint FAO/WHO expert group recommended a daily allowance of 1 mcg of vitamin B_{12} which is lower than the usual recommended dietary intake. This included a large safety factor. So, it is conceivable that some bacteria-laden vegetable foods, such as sprouts and unwashed greens, contain sufficient vitamin B_{12} (e.g. 0.3 mcg) to meet your physiological needs. According to *Vegan Nutrition* (Langley 1988), healthy vegans of up to twenty years' standing, with no obvious source of the vitamin in their diets, will often show a stable blood-serum level of half the minimum level of the accepted range, just above the level considered by physiologists to represent definite deficiency. However, some vegans go below this level and develop serious symptoms.

The non-vegan alternatives are to eat some dairy products (1 cup milk provides nearly 1 mcg vitamin B_{12}), eggs or some lower (less sentient) life forms, such as fish or insects. The dairy products will stimulate the excretion of mucus in your digestive tract, providing a haven for parasites and infections such as the common cold. If you eat eggs you may risk cholesterol build-up (see Eating for the Heart). I currently prefer to eat about 25 g raw (if fresh) fish a day (or 100 g every four days, preferably including the calcium-rich bones from, for example, fish such as sardines or salmon). Pregnant and lactating mothers must take precautions to obtain sufficient vitamin B_{12} to avoid damage to their baby.

The flip side of this is to watch for vitamin or mineral overdose. The obvious way to risk overdose is to take vitamin and mineral pills. A Symbiotic needs no such chemical constructions. If your food is grown in depleted soil or hydroponics, which may be wanting in trace minerals, then vitamin supplements may be necessary. Seaweed would be a better choice because it is a very rich source of minerals in a biological package. Seaweed contains 10 to 50 times as much minerals as vegetables (Hewitt 1964).

The less obvious way to overdose on minerals is by eating in an unbalanced way according to the CaPNaK Chart. For example, an underdose of calcium has symptoms in common with an overdose of phosphorus.

Unfortunately, the insidious scourge of phosphorus poisoning from eating grains (or meat) is officially condoned. The 1990 report, *Healthy People 2000: National Health Promotion and Disease Prevention Objectives*, of the US Department of Health and Human Services recommends that the average total fat intake among people aged two and older be no more than 30 per cent of kilojoules and that the saturated fat intake should not exceed 10 per cent of kilojoules. It also advises the daily consumption of five or more servings of vegetables, fruits and legumes, and six or more servings of grain products.

There is no large Symbiotic community on this planet yet. Unfortunately, the statistical study of the nutritional benefits of a fruit-oriented diet must wait until such a community exists.

A diagram showing the Symbiotic counter-proposal is given on the following page.

The next revolution in consensus nutrition will be the replacement of grain by fruit as the recommended primary food. This will take many years and much suffering by the believers of the growing Macrobiotic mainstream.

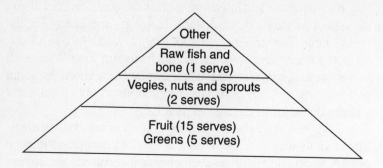

The symbiotic food pyramid: fruit and leafy greens form the basis, the 'other' foods at the apex are eaten in debauched moments, if at all.

Eating for Immunity

Once upon a time a man called Henry longed to own a car. He worked hard and saved his money, and by and by he went to buy a car. Jane, the lady who sold him the car, told him, 'Cars get energy by burning fuel. Just put the fuel in the tank, and off you go.'

When Henry went home he had steak and eggs for dinner. After dinner he decided to put some fuel in the car's tank. So he chopped up some wood and pushed it into the tank. To Henry's dismay, his car wouldn't go. He called Jane, and she said, 'Henry, wood won't pour through the pipes into the engine! Now you'll have to clean out the tank.'

The next morning, Henry ate his breakfast cereal and drank a big glass of milk. After breakfast, he cleaned out the tank, and then he poured in a tinful of kerosene. To Henry's frustration, the car still wouldn't go. He called Jane, and she said, 'Henry, kerosene won't burn in the engine! Wash out the engine, and put petrol in the tank.'

Henry took Jane's advice, but as he tightened the petrol cap he felt sick and exhausted, so he drove off to see his doctor. His doctor said, 'Henry, you're in bad shape. You had better stop eating meat and milk. Eat more fruit and less cooked food. You need a good clean out.'

Henry replied, 'Doctor, I can't stop eating meat and milk and cooked food! My body needs them to burn for energy. If I restrict what I eat, I won't have the energy to look after my car!'

Henry left his car to Jane in his will. She drove it to shop at the greengrocer's for years because Henry had taken such good care of it.

The body-mind has very special fuel requirements to keep it running in optimum health. The food of the human body-mind has symbiotically co-evolved with us humans and our primate ancestors over millions of years. If we eat alien or mutilated (cooked) foods, the immune system of the body-mind valiantly struggles to clean out the collecting debris. However, fat and cholesterol deposit in the circulatory system, uric acid crystallises in the tissues, mucus collects in the digestive tract, and free radicals and oxidised tissues accumulate throughout the body-mind. Eventually, the immune system is overpowered, and disease takes control.

This process is most obvious with the common cold. When dairy products are eaten the body-mind has difficulty breaking down this alien food. Strong digestive juices are excreted in the stomach. Then mucus is excreted in the throat and nose to protect the sensitive mucous membrane from also being attacked by these digestive juices. If dairy products are eaten daily, the mucus stays in the nose and throat. This provides a home for bacterial and viral infection. Eventually the infection gets out of hand, and the immune system calls in the heavy artillery. The result is a cleansing crisis known as the common cold. The preventative of the common cold has been known for years: stop eating dairy products and other mucus-provoking foods!

Detoxifying or cleansing the body-mind through fasting has been strongly emphasised in fruitarian literature. Unfortunately, some irrationalists have propagated the belief that bacteria and viruses have no role in disease. They believe toxins are the only cause of disease, and ludicrously reject the reality of infection (Ehret 1953).

Louis Pasteur did say, on his death bed, that the terrain (the body-mind) is more important than the germ. However, this is not to say that the germ is unimportant: both the germ and the terrain are partners in disease. Public health measures have been, and will continue to be, a very significant factor in preventing the spread of infection.

Besides these gross problems of accumulation, there is a more subtle threat to immunity that lies at the very foundation of our culture of death. That is food mutilation, otherwise euphemistically know as the exquisite art of cuisine.

For millions of years our hominid ancestors lived in the fruit-filled forests of Africa. A few hundred thousand years ago some of them left Africa and wandered into the colder regions of the planet.

About 100 000 years ago someone discovered how to build a fire. Thousands of years later the ice age hit. A cold hunter-gather, frustrated in a search for fruit, found that firing up an animal or grass seeds made them soft and edible.

During the last ice age, which started about 80 000 years ago, others worked out how to make large animals more edible by cooking. The next step was to domesticate cattle to assure a plentiful and mobile supply of meat. However, with so much meat being consumed, our wandering ancestors began to suffer from acidity and the associated calcium deficit. It must have been a desperate moment when a human, hunched by a dissolving spine, first drank milk from a cow.

About 10 000 years ago other sore-footed wanderers decided to settle down and grow cereal. That was a fateful and fatal decision. They could have decided to grow fruit, but probably the need for a short growing cycle, storability and portability dictated their decision. We can forgive these desperate ancestors, but need not continue to be victims of their decisions!

Food mutilation involves heating food to make chemical changes. This creates twisted and alien molecules, which tax the immune system. If treatment of food with heat was a new innovation, government bodies would probably ban the process! Living food contains activated enzymes, specially shaped molecules with delicately distributed electrons. These activated enzymes are biochemical tools that help the body-mind digest the living food. They also help the immune system in cleansing the body-mind.

When you heat a food above 50°C (122°F), you deactivate or destroy these delicate enzymes. The body-mind then has to make up for the shortfall in digestive enzymes by squeezing extra juice from the pancreas. The pancreas is part of the endocrine system, and the endocrine system is the powerhouse of the immune system. A depleted pancreas leads to an unbalanced immune system, reducing the body's ability to cleanse, detoxify, disinfect itself, and destroy cancer cells.

So, if you want optimum immunity, you must stop draining the pancreas of enzymes—by eating more unmutilated food. Complex carbohydrates from cereals and grains are an especially severe drain on pancreatic digestive enzymes, a factor in cancer becoming more prevalent as more people eat more grain. The move from animal foods to grain replaces heart disease with cancer.

Cancer is a scourge of the Japanese, whose immunity is depleted by their rice-eating. Also, their intake of foods of animal origin has more than doubled since 1960. Some cancers associated with meat-eating and other factors have increased in Japan, and since 1980 cancer has become the greatest cause of death (*Asahi Shimbin Japan Almanac* 1993).

If you are obese you are more susceptible to a wide range of bacterial infections and cancers. A high-fat intake can speed up the shrinking of your thymus, which is responsible for programming your immune cells (Berger 1985).

Food allergies are a widespread and unrecognised problem for immunity. Everyone has their own individual food allergies. Blood tests (cytotoxic testing) will determine your allergenic foods. When you eat your allergenic foods they kill or damage many of your white blood cells, depleting your immune system of its defences; when your immune cells are exposed to the toxins from certain allergenic foods, they swell up and explode! If your immune system becomes weakened you will slowly grow more sluggish, start losing vitality, energy and sexual drive. The ageing process is accelerated, resulting in premature wrinkles and skin problems.

You can help your immune system by reducing your intake of your allergenic substances (allergens). You can also help your immune system to strengthen its defences. Allergens, bacteria, yeast and other toxins that enter your bloodstream mostly consist of protein. These proteins can be digested by enzymes in your bloodstream (Santillo 1987). You can increase the amount of enzymes available in your bloodstream by reducing the demand for enzymes in your digestive tract. When you eat live fruit and vegetables, enzymes in the food help your digestion. Then your digestion of the food is more complete, and undigested food proteins do not enter your bloodstream. You win both ways: better digestion and stronger immunity, or put another way, fewer allergens and more enzymes.

Medical scientists have been puzzled by the fact that

most people have hidden food sensitivities to the very foods that appear most nourishing and healthy. Allergies to wheat, corn, and dairy products are so common that at least one of these afflicts almost every American. Yeast, sugar, coffee, eggs, and soy products are also common villains (Berger, 1985).

You can see their dilemma: they have recently accepted that meat should be substantially replaced with cereals and legumes, and then they collide with the problem of allergies and depressed immunity resulting from cereals and legumes! Of course humans react to these foods as if they were invaders: they are not fit (evolved) for human (primate) consumption! The solution to the puzzle is fruit, but that is just too difficult for some to accept since it involves too much intellectual reprogramming and too many life-style changes.

You can restore your immunity by eliminating your allergenic foods and ensuring you get the amino acids, vitamins and minerals for rebuilding your immune system. Your body builds 200 000 new immune cells every second of your life, and your food is an essential supplier of the raw materials for their construction. If you destroy immune cells at a faster rate than you construct them, as a result of eating foods to which you are allergic, then you will crave too much food and get fatter—especially if you eat low-nutrition foods, which do not provide the desperately needed raw materials for building immune cells. Alternatively, when your immune system becomes strong and stable, your eating patterns become more established, and you get and stay thinner.

You can find out which foods you are allergic to by first eliminating the seven most toxic foods for twenty-one days. You may experience withdrawal symptoms in the first week of elimination, during which time your immune system freaks out, wondering why you are suddenly being so kind to it.

According to Berger (1985), the seven most toxic foods are:

- cow's milk products
- wheat
- yeast

- eggs
- corn
- soy products
- cane sugar.

Then (just for kicks) reintroduce these foods one at a time to threaten your immune system. Every second day eat one of the seven foods three times. Listen to your body-mind to observe the degree to which you react to each of these foods. You will know you have done the wrong thing if you wake up in the middle of the night and hear your immune system moaning 'Oh no, not that again!' Other common symptoms of a food allergy are fatigue, anxiety, depression, tension, headaches, and more obvious physical conditions such as skin problems. Don't bother reintroducing them to your usual eating patterns: save them for especially debauched moments. Food allergy experts suggest eating toxic foods *no more than once every four days*, if at all.

People usually binge on exactly the foods to which they have allergies. Bingeing releases a type of hormone called beta-endorphines, which are the body-mind's own opiate substances. This gives the binger a high similar to those that athletes can experience, and explains the addictive quality of bingeing. A food binge works like a safety valve to relieve anxiety momentarily. Some healthier alternative method of relieving stress and anxiety, such as exercise or meditation, is more productive. Guided imagery can create a positive mental attitude that influences your body-mind chemistry to strengthen your immune system. For example, close your eyes and imagine yourself successfully dealing with the stressful situations with a relaxed, positive attitude.

Food allergies can also create emotional disturbances, such as depression, hyperactivity, anxiety, irritability and aggressive behaviour.

Eating for the Heart

You cannot get more central than the heart, the whole body-mind depends on it for life. The heart keeps itself alive by pumping blood through its own coronary arteries. An American doctor saved his own life when his heart went into fibrillation (unco-ordinated spasms). He deliberately coughed every two seconds until he reached hospital. His coughing pumped enough blood to stop him from losing consciousness! No one can cough their way through life, so it is wise to help your heart take care of itself.

The blockage of these coronary arteries by deposits of plaque on the inner walls of the arteries is a major cause of death. Plaque consists of deposited low-density lipoprotein (LDL) cholesterol and fat. LDL-cholesterol exists naturally in the body, but a high-cholesterol diet supplies excessive LDL-cholesterol to the body-mind. Nevertheless, food cholesterol alone does not result in increased LDL-cholesterol levels in the blood. Saturated fat (animal fat) is a more important factor than food cholesterol in increasing LDL-cholesterol levels in the blood. Higher blood-levels of LDL-cholesterol are associated with the build-up of plaque in the arteries.

The body-mind tries to remove the plaques with its garbage-collecting cells called macrophages. However, if there is too much to collect, the macrophages explode because they become over-loaded with LDL-cholesterol. Then, free radicals released from exploded macrophages oxidise the cholesterol in the plaque. Unfortunately, macrophages cannot mop up oxidised cholesterol. So the plaque continues to accumulate until it blocks an artery. If it happens to be a coronary artery—heart attack!

Eating rancid fats also leads to high levels of free radicals, which may reinforce the damage. It is very important to eat fresh, un-oxidised, sources of fat. This includes nut butters such as tahini; replace these with whole, fresh seeds and nuts if there is any risk of rancidity.

In the 1970s health pioneer Nathan Pritikin showed people how to significantly reduce LDL-cholesterol levels. His method was a very low-cholesterol and low-fat diet, combined with an aerobic exercise programme (Horne 1985).

Mono-unsaturated fat is the only fat that does not have a bad reputation. It raises the levels of HDL-cholesterol, and HDL-cholesterol protects against heart disease. See Eating for Weight Gain for more information about mono-unsaturated fat. Any person interested in basic health must work towards a low-fat approach to low-cholesteral eating.

Here are some informative statistics:

Risk of death from heart attack for the average man on a Western diet	50%
Risk of death from heart attack for the average man who consumes no meat	15%
Risk of death from heart attack for the average man who consumes no meat, dairy products or eggs	4%
Rise in blood cholesterol from consuming 1 egg per day	12%
Rise in heart-attack risk from 12% rise in blood cholesterol	24%

(EarthSave Foundation 1992)

High-sodium eating habits are associated with heart disease, and high-potassium eating has been found to reduce blood pressure. Use the CaPNaK Chart to learn which foods have a sodium- or potassium-residue, and reduce your risk of cardiovascular diseases. Remember that sodium (salt) is added to many processed foods; they should be avoided.

Exercise does not burn up cholesterol. Many meat-eating joggers have died thinking they were safe from cholesterol build-up. Exercise burns fat, but not cholesterol.

Eating for the Teeth

Fruit sugar comes with natural antibiotics and enzymes that discourage but do not completely prevent tooth decay. I recommend daily brushing, flossing and regular dental checkups. From my personal experience, I can say there is no guarantee that a fruit diet will prevent tooth decay. Perhaps, if I had always been eating 750 g green-leaf vegetables daily, I would have had even fewer tooth problems.

On a more positive note, I completely reversed receding gums and abscesses by eating such large quantities of green-leaf vegetables. Two dentists had told me to have root therapy for a tooth under which I had an abscess. However, after three years without treatment I now have no symptoms of the abscess, and no sensitivity or bleeding from receding gums after I brush my teeth. Now my dentist cannot believe that I ever had an abscess.

Receding gums should be taken as an early warning of calcium deficiency or phosphorus overdose, and potential osteoporosis. The jaw-bone around the teeth is one of the first places the body-mind draws calcium from when there is a deficit; the gum then recedes, following the underlying bone. This imbalance can be corrected using the CaPNaK Chart. By creating receding gums, nature makes the teeth sensitive. This discourages the eater from eating hard seeds and nuts. Otherwise, too many seeds and nuts would leave a high phosphorus-residue in the body-mind and make the problem worse. When the calcium–phosphorus balance is restored, calcium is absorbed back into the jaw-bone, and the gums grow back to normal.

A toothless frugivorous man once told me that having no teeth is a privileged higher stage of evolution for divine beings who only eat soft fruit! The problem is, though, that every grin becomes a laugh.

Eating for Weight Loss

In our society, if you are significantly overfat you are probably unhappy, with feelings of guilt and shame about being out of control of your body, resentment, loneliness, and real or imagined sexual inadequacy.

Overfat people get sick more often, and suffer more headaches, joint pain, stomach upsets, and skin problems. They are more prone to depression, mood swings, fatigue and lethargy. They age faster, are more prone to degenerative diseases like diabetes, cancer and heart disease, and they have less energy and stamina.

It has been reported that about 48 per cent of men and 33 per cent of women are overfat, and 94 per cent of women want to be slimmer (of these 20 per cent use laxatives or vomiting, 17 per cent binge at least once a week) (Mulham 1995).

Some people cannot lose weight on 5000 kilojoules a day, and some cannot gain on 13 000 kilojoules a day. In other words, some people can eat huge meals and not become fat, while others become fat on meagre diets. This difference is partly inherited, but there are also physiological and psychological factors that are a result of the individual's life experience and behaviour.

One important factor is the acid–alkaline balance of the body-mind. Alkalinity and the related availability of calcium makes fat absorption from the intestine easier. Many people who are overfat have thick, dense bones, full of calcium. This may be partly due to a high intake of dairy products during childhood and adolescence. These people absorb fats very easily. If such alkaline people then go on a classic low-kilojoule, fat-loss diet, they actually worsen their problem. This is because such diets, emphasising large salads with low-fat cheese and yogurt, add even more calcium to their body-mind. When they return to balanced eating, their increased alkalinity assures resumed fat gain.

If you want to lose fat, then you must eat low-kilojoule foods that also increase the acidity of the body-mind. Experiments have shown that a higher intake of phosphorus (acidic) depresses appetite and weight gain of adult rats and pigs (Draper & Scythes 1981). To create this effect in your own body-mind, you must emphasise fruit and vegetables in your diet to give a phosphorus-residue (with the exception of avocado). In other words, by moving away from the CaPNaK balance point and eating more acid foods, you can reduce the absorption of fats by your body-mind.

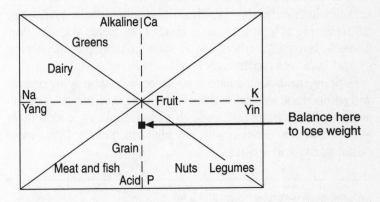

Change body fat by using a shifted balance point on the CaPNaK Chart.

You must also avoid fatty food, especially in combination with calcium-residue foods. Thus, dairy products, especially cheese, are for high debauchery only. Cottage cheese is an exception, since it is a phosphorus-residue food in the yang–acid quadrant of the CaPNaK Chart. It may take several years until you reduce your alkalinity to a point where, even with balanced eating, you do not gain fat. This depends on the initial degree of alkalinity of your body-mind.

Another advantage of eating more phosphorus-residue foods is that the level of arousal and anxiety of the body-mind will increase (refer to the symptoms of phosphorus overdose on page 19). This will result in increased mental and physical activity levels, which will help burn kilojoules. This fight-and-flight response can be positive, provided it is not excessive. It especially benefits those overfat people who tend to be less active.

However, if you have any symptoms of low bone-mineral density or calcium depletion, then you must be more cautious. Eat at least 750 g green-leaf vegetables daily to provide adequate calcium. In that case, fruit-oriented eating around the CaPNaK balance point will lead to fat loss.

It is important to think thin: never drive if you can pedal or walk somewhere. If you work in an office, always take a walk at lunchtime. Drop the lifestyle of three meals a day: just graze throughout the day. Meals load up the bloodstream with carbohydrate (blood sugar), which stimulates the release of insulin. Insulin helps store fat, so having at least six smaller feeds a day helps you stay thin. Recent research (Waterhouse 1993) shows snacking reduces obesity and improves blood-sugar levels.

Skipping meals, doing little or no exercise, and bingeing on fatty and refined food slows down the fat-burning metabolism. You can increase your metabolism through exercise and by eating more often. However, exercise with too high an intensity burns more carbohydrate and less fat.

Running   (20 minutes) burns 2.9 g fat

Jogging   (30 minutes) burns 5.3 g

Aerobics   (45 minutes) burns 10 g

Walking   (60 minutes) burns 17.8 g

(Mulham 1995)

Exercise producing a pulse rate of 120 beats a minute (20 beats in 10 seconds) is best for burning fat. Slow down if you get puffed, turn red, or feel faint.

The following table shows how more frequent eating increases metabolism (Basal Metabolic Rate—BMR), enabling faster fat loss. Each row of the table shows a different eating schedule.

Breakfast	Snack	Lunch	Snack	Dinner	Snack	Change in BMR	
No	No	No	No	Yes	No	−5.9%	Slows down BMR; weight gain
No	No	Yes	No	Yes	No	−4.9%	
Small	No	Yes	No	Yes	No	−2.4%	
Yes	No	Yes	No	Yes	No	0%	Speeds up BMR; weight loss
Yes	Yes	Yes	Yes	Yes	No	+1.4%	
Yes	Yes	Yes	Yes	Yes	Yes	+3.1%	

(Mulham 1995)

You can also speed up your metabolism by eating spices such as chillies and ginger. Eat smaller meals at night when your metabolism is low, otherwise you will convert excess food to body fat.

To avoid the confusion about the word 'diet', I have used 'diet' to mean what you usually eat, and 'dieting' to mean reducing your kilojoule intake.

You 'turn on' your fat cells by dieting or fasting for 72 hours: lipogenic (fat-storing) enzymes are activated, and lipolytic (fat-burning) enzymes are deactivated. You then store more fat after the dieting because your fat cells stay turned on. Also, you lose kilojoule-burning muscle during dieting. So your ratio of fat to muscle is increased after dieting. Your fat cells can also be turned on by overeating: fat cells divide into two when they get too big, so you end up with more fat cells after overeating.

Smaller, more numerous, low-fat meals turn off your fat cells by deactivating your lipogenic enzymes. Regular, moderate aerobic exercise is the way to activate your lipolytic (fat-burning) enzymes. You must exercise continuously for about 30 minutes to begin to activate your lipolytic enzymes. Exercise beyond 30 minutes burns fat faster, so a minimum of 45 minutes is preferable—at least three times a week. If you exercise too hard, you reduce the oxygen available to burn fat (Waterhouse 1993).

Women tend to be fatter than men because oestrogen stimulates the release of lipogenic (fat-storing) enzymes. When a woman enters menopause her oestrogen level reduces. However, rather than losing body fat, fat tends to redistribute to her waist. Her metabolic rate also decreases by about 10 per cent, so she doesn't need to eat as much (Waterhouse 1993). If your body fat increases more than you want during menopause, slightly increase your exercise activities, and eat even more lightly and more often.

Beware of hidden sources of fat. Meat eaters should note that a takeaway hamburger could contain up to 31 g fat. The highest sources of fat in the symbiotic's menu are nuts and seeds, which contain about 59 g fat per 100 g.

Fatty tissue in obese people is deficient in lipase. Lipase is an enzyme that aids the breaking down of stored fats. You can get lipase from live, unheated food.

Fatty tissue also provides storage space for toxic wastes in the body-mind. Detoxification progresses with the cleansing provoked by living food. Eventually, the body-mind no longer needs toxic waste storage space, and then this fat is removed.

If you want to lose fat, you must understand the process, change your lifestyle, and set realistic and achievable goals of slow, but permanent, fat loss. If you are overfat and sedentary, you have about twice the risk of dying from a heart attack. You are also more likely to be robbed of years of your life by heart disease, cancer, stroke, diabetes, gallbladder disease, or joint problems. Appearance is not the only reason to lose fat!

Eating for Weight Gain

R ead the reasoning about the relationship between acidity and fat loss in Eating for Weight Loss. By reversing the reasoning, it makes sense that many people who are underfat have thin, light bones bereft of calcium. This is often due to a low intake of dairy products or green-leaf vegetables during childhood and adolescence. These people lose fat very easily.

If such acid people then go on a classic high-kilojoule, fat-gain diet emphasising meat, grain, legumes and nuts, they actually worsen their problem. Such foods add acidity, and rob even more calcium from their bones. When they return to balanced eating, their acidity assures resumed fat loss.

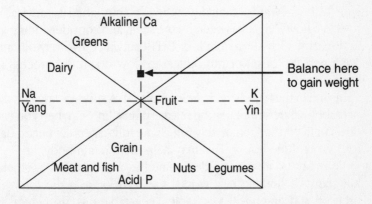

Change body fat by using a shifted balance point on the CaPNaK Chart.

By emphasising the eating of alkaline foods you can absorb fat more easily. However, it may take several years to reduce the acidity of the body-mind so it can retain the fat. You must note that natural sources of fat, such as nuts, seeds and avocados are phosphorus-residue foods. This means that the body-mind will not absorb their fat easily unless you combine them with enough calcium-residue foods, such as green-leaf vegetables. Refer to the CaPNaK Chart.

Nuts with green-leaf vegetables provide an acid–alkaline balance for building up tissues. The acidity of nuts requires that they be eaten in very small quantities: an upper daily limit is about 10 g nuts for every 100 g green-leaf vegetables; 10 g nuts daily is the minimum. Nuts and seeds are a good source of the amino acid, arginine, which stimulates the release of growth hormone from the pituitary gland. Growth hormone stimulates muscle growth, which is a useful way to gain weight.

One source of vegetable fat providing a calcium-residue is unhulled sesame seeds, or the sesame paste known as unhulled tahini. However, please note that hulled sesame seeds and hulled tahini are very acidic. Both hulled and unhulled sesame seeds are shown on the CaPNaK Chart. Note the enormous acid–alkaline difference between them! Unhulled tahini has 600 mg of calcium per 100 g, whereas hulled tahini has only 14 mg per 100 g. Unhulled tahini is a very useful dressing or dip for live foods, and can help you gain fat, but beware of rancidity. When you buy tahini it is advisable to check how long it has been on the shelf, and consider adding an antioxidant such as vitamin E or BHT (butylated hydroxytoluene; 1 tsp per litre of oil or nut butter) to slow down the process of rancidity.

Insulin in the bloodstream helps store fat. A sudden, large intake of carbohydrate stimulates the release of insulin. So, when you eat, do so until you are completely full. Some fruit-eaters eat once a day for two or three hours. This may help them retain body fat.

You may be absolutely determined to put on a few aesthetic kilograms. If nothing else works, use olive oil as a dip for your broccoli and green-leaf vegetables; vegetable oils are neutral in their acid–alkaline balance. If necessary, I can put on half a kilogram a week by consuming daily 100 g olive oil with calcium-residue foods. This practice is destructively unhealthy, and should not be continued over a long period. However, olive oil or other mono-unsaturated fats are a healthier choice than polyunsaturated fats and oils because they are less reactive with tissue. Olives, avocados and cashews are good sources of mono-unsaturated fat. Polyunsaturated fats and oils contribute to cancer, even when they are slightly rancid. Rancidity is harder to smell in polyunsaturated oils, so store these fats and oils, in sealed containers, in the refrigerator. Saturated fats can deposit in the arteries, and contribute to heart disease.

Limit yourself to no more than 7.5 per cent of your daily kilojoules from polyunsaturated sources such as nuts, no more than 7.5 per cent from saturated fats from animal sources, and no more than 15 per cent from mono-unsaturated sources (Pearson & Shaw 1982). However, these standards are set on the high side because they allow 30 per cent of kilojoules to be fats. A healthier standard would be for between 10 and 20 per cent of kilojoules to be fats—Pritikin stipulated 10 per cent (Pritikin & McGrady 1973). You may understand by now that healthier goals are austere only when stodgy grain is recommended as the staple, rather than fruit!

We live in a culture that expects people to carry significant amounts of fat, a result of the high-fat, high-kilojoule Western diet. It is natural to be thin; wild animals are thin, unless they live in a very cold climate and the majority of people on this planet are thin. So, if you are thin and wish to attain a conventionally expected weight, it is likely you will have to eat unnatural foods such as oil, cooked grain and meat, or dairy products. I prefer to stay a little under the conventionally expected weight for my height. I know one Symbiotic who retains weight by eating large quantities of raw fish; however, he is facing the risks of increased acidity from the high phosphorus-residue of fish.

Excessive fat loss indicates that you may not be eating enough calcium-residue foods. If you are an acidic, hyperactive, super-thin person, these foods will calm you down and reduce your tendency to burn yourself up with activities. Rest and digest.

Idealistic people who practise pure fruitarianism (eating fruit only) become super-thin partly because of low calcium intake. Through their enlightenment they will precede us to Paradise. All rigid ideals have a paradox rushing towards them—the paradox of pure fruitarianism is osteoporosis.

Eating for Cooling

T he skin is your cooling system. You can turn it on or off using the sodium-potassium residue dimension of the CaPNaK Chart. For cooling, the idea is to increase blood circulation near the skin, and increase blood volume, by using high sodium-residue (yang) foods. This increases convection cooling with the air and evaporative cooling from perspiration.

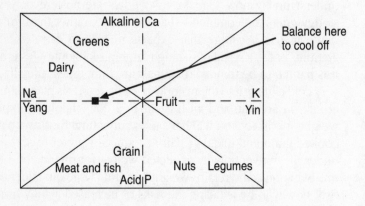

Yang: warmth and expansion outside, coolness and contraction inside.

Try it for yourself. For example, buy a bunch of celery, and eat six stalks during an afternoon. You will feel particularly cool or cold in the evening, because celery is one of the highest vegetable sources of sodium-residue. Kelp (seaweed) is even higher in sodium-residue, but you must acquire the taste for it. I collect it from the beach, rinse it in seawater, cut it into short strips, sun-dry them, and store them in a sealed jar. Kelp is in the yang–alkaline (top left-hand) corner of the CaPNaK Chart. It is ten to fifty times more yang than celery, and must be eaten in proportionately smaller amounts.

If you are at the ocean, drink a little seawater to cool off. Seawater has a sodium-residue. Drinking seawater in small amounts was advised by Hippocrates. It is a source of a wide range of minerals.

To ensure you get enough calcium, choose high sodium- and calcium-residue green-leaf vegetables, such as spinach, during hot weather. Mangoes are one of the best fruits for sodium-residue because they have one of the lowest potassium-residues of all fruit (see the CaPNaKChart).

As a Symbiotic you must consider the timing of eating sodium-residue foods during the day to regulate cooling of the body-mind. It is best to eat the largest quantity of sodium-residue foods around midday when the temperature is highest. Beware of eating a high-sodium-residue meal such as a large salad or Chinese mixed vegetables on a cold winter evening.

Darker skin absorbs heat out of the body-mind and convects and radiates it away. That is why your skin darkens with suntanning. It is cooler to have a dark skin, but do not overdo it. Thirty minutes of sunshine a day is enough, but if you are prone to skin cancer you may need to limit your exposure even more.

Eating for Warmth

For warming, the idea is to decrease blood circulation near the skin, and decrease blood volume, by eating high potassium-residue (yin) foods. This reduces convection cooling to the air and evaporative cooling from perspiration.

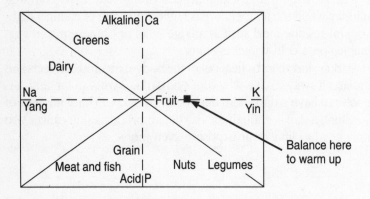

Yin: coolness and contraction outside, warmth and expansion inside.

Again, try it for yourself. For example, buy a bunch of bananas, and eat five bananas during a morning. You should feel particularly warm or hot by around midday, because bananas are high in potassium-residue. Pumpkin, tomato and dates are also high in potassium-residue.

To get warm, avoid high sodium-residue foods, but make sure you get enough calcium. For your green vegetables, choose the potassium-residue, high-calcium-residue greens, such as broccoli, during cold weather (see the CaPNaK Chart).

When you are warm enough, it is wise to eat some sodium-residue foods. For example, three sticks of celery a day will supply your minimum sodium requirements.

As a Symbiotic, you must consider the timing of eating your potassium-residue foods during the day to regulate warming of the body-mind. It is best to eat the largest quantity of potassium-residue foods in the morning and evening when the temperature is lowest. Beware of eating a high-potassium-residue meal, such as too many bananas or pumpkin soup, on a hot summer day. In warm weather two or three bananas a day is enough, while in cool weather five or six should be adequate.

Light skin reflects heat back into the body-mind, so if you have light skin you will be more comfortable in a cooler climate. Many Symbiotics live happily in a temperate climate. If the cold remains a problem despite the use of potassium-residue foods, try warming your food to 50°C (120°F) by steaming, or from sunshine. Higher temperatures will mutilate your food. Do not keep fruit or vegetables in a refrigerator, if possible, because eating cold fruit and vegetables during cool weather is not invigorating. Wear more layers of clothes, with the inner layer being white.

If you really want to get a fire burning within you, you might consider overdosing on phosphorus-residue foods for several decades. If you can deposit sufficient phosphorus in your body, you might just depart by spontaneous combustion.

Eating for Longevity

In what thou eatest and drinkest, seeking from thence
Due nourishment, not gluttonous delight,
Till many years over thy head return:
So maist thou live, till like ripe Fruit, thou drop
Into thy mother's lap; or be with ease
Gatherd, not harshly pluckt, for death mature.
—Milton, *Paradise Lost*, XI*

What are you going to do when you die? Go to Paradise, reincarnate, compost, or increase in entropy? Whichever you believe, there is a reasonable chance that you are enjoying living right now, especially if you are a Symbiotic. In that case, longevity may be an appealing possibility. Many people have sought the virtue of longevity. Three modern examples are instructive: Nathan Pritikin, Professor Arnold Ehret and Dr Norman Walker. All three are dead. If only dead nutrition experts could rewrite their books!

During the 1970s Pritikin made a great contribution to the cause of health and longevity with the *Pritikin Program for Diet and Exercise* (Pritikin & McGrady 1973). He advocated eating mostly complex carbohydrates, and drastically reducing the intake of cholesterol, fat, and protein. He cured himself and many others of cardiovascular disease, but at the pinnacle of his success he died of leukaemia. For the reasons why a high intake of mutilated grain-based food may be associated with leukaemia, see Eating for Immunity.

---

* *Complete Poetry and Selected Prose of John Milton*, Random House, New York, 1950, p. 365.

Ehret was well known in Europe early this century for his long fasts and for his healing through food (Ehret 1953). He advocated a diet of fruit and green-leaf vegetables, and appeared to be in extraordinary health. He emphasised fruit far more than green-leaf vegetables, and often ate only fruit. In 1922 at the pinnacle of his success at the age of 56, after giving a public lecture in Los Angeles, he died from a fractured skull after falling backwards while crossing a road. Now, one can only wonder at the condition of his bones. I suspect that his decades of low-calcium intake dissolved them away. Otherwise, slipping over rarely has such terminal results (see Eating for Bone and Soft Tissue).

Norman Walker was a nutritionist and author, and was well known in the USA for his electric juicers. He advocated eating fruit and large quantities of vegetables, often as juice cocktails. After curing himself of a terminal illness in his thirties, he lived to be 109 years old! He died one morning in 1985 while working in his study. Maybe while he was trying to work out what he would eat at his 110th birthday party? Private correspondence on Walker from his publisher, Norwalk Press, indicates he was healthy up until his death.

The message is clear to me. Norman Walker came closest to the optimum. We can attain longevity by eating fruit and large quantities of raw vegetables (Walker 1949). Vegetables offer certain minerals, such as calcium, in concentrations unavailable in fruit. This is especially so with green-leaf vegetables. I suggest that you should eat at least 750 g a day.

There is also medical evidence:

frequent consumption of vegetables and fruits, especially green and yellow vegetables and citrus fruits, is associated with decreased susceptibility to cancers of the lung, stomach, and large intestine. The mechanism is unknown but it may be related to the carotenoid or dietary fibre content of these foods or to various other nutritive and nonnutritive components. (Thomas 1991)

Fruit and vegetables contain natural preservatives called antioxidants. Antioxidants play a role of major importance in preventing the random damage of ageing that results largely from oxidants in the body. Uncontrolled oxidants such as free radicals 'burn up' tissue, and are the enemy of life-giving enzymes. In electrical terms, free radicals electrocute cells and molecules, and antioxidants short-circuit free radicals.

You can get an idea of the damage already done to your body-mind using the skin-pinch test. Place one hand palm down on a table, and take a fold of skin at the back of the hand, and pull it up taut. Hold it for five seconds, then release it and time how long the skin takes to return to its normal position. Young skin snaps back. The more cross-linking damage you have from oxidants, including free radicals, the more slowly your skin recovers.

Oxidation of foods, especially fats and oils, produces chemicals that are mutagenic (mutation-causing), carcinogenic (cancer-causing), immuno-suppressive and clot-promoting (Pearson & Shaw 1982). The more fat you eat—especially the unsaturated type —the more free radicals your body makes. Free radicals interact with unsaturated fats to produce even more free radicals. This and normal oxidation lead to rancidity.

These are some of the reasons why free fats and oils are such a health risk, especially oily 'health foods' that do not contain antioxidants. If you want to eat oils, buy antioxidants such as BHT (butylated hydroxytoluene) or ascorbyl palmitate for mixing with the oils to reduce free-radical formation, or buy oils containing antioxidants. The choice is simple: rancidity or longevity.

Vitamins C and E are antioxidants. Some antioxidant foods, high in vitamin E, are asparagus, beet green, broccoli, and sweet potato. Further antioxidant foods high in vitamin C are black currant, citrus fruit, collard green, papaya, peppers, potato, strawberry, tomato and watercress. Brussels sprout, spinach and turnip green are good sources of both vitamins C and E. Other antioxidant vitamins and minerals are well supplied by raw fruit and vegetables. However, vitamin C is destroyed by heat and oxygen, vitamin E by freezing.

To summarise the principles of eating for longevity: eat foods low in fat, cholesterol, phosphorus- and sodium-residues; the food should also be high in enzymes. To reduce digestive stress, and improve elimination, minimal kilojoules should be eaten (under-nutrition, not malnutrition). A 6300–8500 kilojoules/day diet should result in additional longevity of 10–40 years, depending how early in life you start! Such undernutrition is easy and satisfying when you eat fruit and green-leaf vegetables.

Those foods near the edge of the CaPNaK Chart are extreme foods. These extreme foods have a very high residue of one or two of the CaPNaK minerals, so they easily throw you out of CaPNaK balance. To reduce physiological stress you are wise to maintain a subtle CaPNaK balance by eating small quantities, rather than eating large quantities of the extreme foods.

It is worth knowing your blood-chemistry profile to screen yourself for diet-related illnesses, such as diabetes, gout, liver disease, and kidney and heart problems. The earlier you know you have a problem the more effective will be your responses. Drink only water for twelve hours before the appropriate blood test. Ask your doctor for a copy of the analysis, which will include the following.

	Unfit mg % (mm/L)	Fit mg % (mm/L)
Total cholesterol	> 200 (5.10)	< 150 (3.85)
HDL-cholesterol	< 30 (0.8)	> 65 (1.7)
Triglycerides	> 150 (1.65)	< 75 (0.82)
Glucose	> 100 (5.5)	< 85 (4.7)
Uric acid: men	> 6 (0.35)	< 4 (0.24)
women	> 7 (0.41)	< 5 (0.30)

(Haas 1983)

When you reach the fit range for these blood factors, you can count yourself among the ultra-healthy.

To show you the spectrum of longevity choices, here are the food chakras (see Eating for Evolution of Consciousness) with corresponding average-life expectancies. These life expectancies are for hypothetical groups of people who eat mainly at the same level throughout their lives.

Chakra	Name	Maximum life-span (years)
7	Symbiotic	120
6	Vegan	110
5	Macrobiotic	100
4	Vegetarian	90
3	Piscavore	80
2	Carnivore	70
1	Junkivore	60

In Tokyo I once attended a lecture by Michio Kushi, one of the founders of Macrobiotics. He had spoken about how Macrobiotics eliminates all diseases and bodily deterioration. So I asked him, 'When everyone on Earth is eating according to Macrobiotics what will people die of?' He hesitated a moment, then leaned towards me, saying under his breath 'Suicide!' Maybe he is right; the gut-grinding stodginess of Macrobiotics probably does lead to suicide! At least one person has died after eating, for an extended period, Macrobiotic Diet Number Seven—the infamous all-brown-rice diet.

The Hunzas are one of the societies in which people often live longer than a century. This is partly because the water they use comes from glaciers, and carries colloidal minerals. Flanagan Technologies (in Arizona) have invented a special powder that forms a colloid in water, which has similar properties to Hunza water. This water has very low surface-tension, and is conducive to biological activity.

People who regularly drink water-based beverages would probably benefit from this kind of water. Symbiotics who get most of their water from live food probably get enough colloids from their food. However, this is a new aspect of nutrition that may become more important for longevity.

Eating for the Climate

It is preferable to eat mostly fruit, vegetables and nuts grown in your climatic zone. Those foods have symbiotically evolved with the animals that eat them. They provide optimum nutrition for your climate.

You may live in a temperate climate where bananas and avocados, for example, do not grow. I do not intend to suggest that you stop eating bananas and avocados; they can be very beneficial and satisfying foods in cold weather. The symbiotic basis for human eating can only be fully applied in a subtropical or tropical climate. Human migration into temperate zones was probably too recent for our food to evolve symbiotically in these zones. So in temperate climates it is usually necessary to eat some fruits that grow in warmer regions, especially the fruit of the subtropical winter.

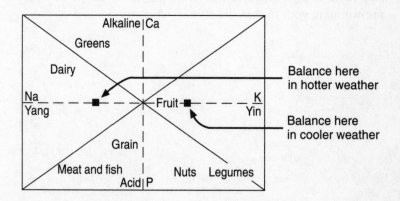

Climatic shifting of the CaPNaK balance point.

The central balance point of the CaPNaK Chart is positioned approximately for a subtropical climate. In colder climates the balance point shifts to approximately the position of the apple on the chart, in the potassium-residue direction. Similarly, in warmer climates the body needs more sodium and extracellular fluid for cooling, so the central balance point of the chart shifts an equal distance in the sodium-residue direction.

People often say that they cannot eat mostly fruit when they live in a temperate climate. This is not so. It is just a matter of being careful about which fruits and vegetables you eat, and when you eat them. For example, it would be a mistake to eat a sodium-residue salad on a cold evening. Beware of salted nuts, seeds, and dressings because the salt is very cooling. Most fruits are quite warming due to their potassium residue. It is not the fruit that makes you cold: it is the sodium-residue vegetables (and salty additives) eaten in the evening. In a temperate climate you should eat sodium-residue vegetables only at midday.

In a temperate zone there are many delicious fruit to choose from: pears, apples, citrus fruits, figs, grapes, plums, berries, bananas, etc.—what you eat doesn't have to be grown in a temperate climate. In winter citrus fruit, avocados, bananas and fruit from cold-storage are all available. A Symbiotic can eat very satisfactorily if a good range of fruit is available. On sunny days, try pre-warming your fruit in the sun.

Eating for the Seasons

Nature provides the appropriate fruits and vegetables according to the seasons in the region where you live. There is a simple reason for this: symbiosis. If the plant feeds you well according to the seasons, the healthier you will be. The more you are attracted by the plant, the more you will spread its seeds and fertilise its soil. At least, that's how it was before civilisation separated us from nature.

It is now time for all Symbiotics to reconnect with Gaia, the Earth Mother, by eating what she provides when she provides it. Tune your eating into the seasons. Eat more bananas, dates, prunes, avocados and pumpkins for warming in winter weather. In summer eat more greens for cooling and carotene (nature's sunscreen), and more melons for water. Don't worry too much about eating locally grown fruit, especially if you live in a temperate zone—humans are an imported species there, so importing some fruit is acceptable.

Again, the central balance point of the CaPNaK Chart shifts with the seasons. The balance point shifts to approximately the position of the apple in the potassium-residue direction in the winter, and an equal distance in the sodium-residue direction in the summer. It is not surprising that pumpkin soup is a popular dish for cold winter days. See Eating for Cooling and Eating for Warmth for more information.

It is very important to eat fruit at room temperature rather than straight from a refrigerator. That way you avoid using your bio-energy to warm up the food. Also, the precious enzymes in the fruit will be active at room temperature. If possible, energise the fruit with sunlight before you eat it. Fruits are intricate translucent organic crystals that, ideally, hang from trees absorbing sunlight and transforming it into vibrant bio-energy, just for you!

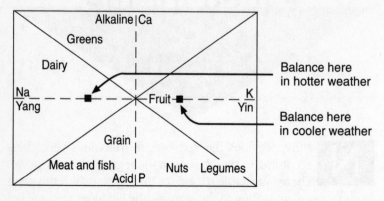

Seasonal shifting of the CaPNaK balance point.

Proverbially speaking, you all know variety is the spice of life, and absence makes the heart grow fonder. In relation to living foods that means that eating seasonally is the way to go. For example, I avoid the exotic avocados available in summer; when the new-season avocados hit the shelves they are a wonderfully fresh taste sensation. This way it is impossible to become bored with living foods. Seasonal variation in eating patterns is also important, to avoid creating allergies from overdosing on a small set of foods. Besides, it is easier on the wallet to eat what is in season.

Below is a list according to the seasons of some of the living foods available in a subtropical climate.

Spring:	apricot, papaya, pineapple, strawberry, tomato.
Summer:	blueberry, celery, grape, mango, melon, nectarine, peach, plum.
Autumn:	apple, avocado, kiwi fruit, orange, pear.
Winter:	apple, avocado, banana, broccoli, citrus, pear, pumpkin.

While particularly useful in winter, bananas are available virtually all year. Use them as a warming and satisfying food for cool subtropical spring and autumn days, or long cool summer nights.

In a temperate climate tropical summer fruits such as papaya and mango may not always be available, but there is usually a range of temperate fruit (pears, apples, nectarines, etc.). Bananas are a warming fruit in temperate zones, irrespective of their origin.

Eating for the Spirit

A subtly balanced diet cannot be maintained by an unstable mind. External and internal life must be brought into order by drawing on the source of infinite light–love–life. Take time out to do what you know you need to do to refill your heart with love. Then subtle diet will just be one aspect of an ever more harmonious life.

Loving inspiration often comes to people through prayer or meditation, but may also come through contemplation, work, play, physical activity, creativity, relationships, or just doing nothing. Each of us knows what spiritual practice is best for us and our particular spectrum of consciousness.

Trying to impose a more refined eating behaviour on oneself or others without spiritual preparation will result in suffering. This will generate inner or outer conflict, and reinforce the illusion of separation—a view of reality that is transcended by a view that sees the oneness of every thing. We know in our hearts that love-compassion is the glue that bonds the parts and creates the wholeness.

Use the CaPNaK Chart to help rebalance your eating, and thereby reduce any psychophysical imbalance. Remain aware that spiritual fulfilment requires development of awareness and activity in all aspects of life, well beyond food.

Three basic aspects of life are your relation to money, food and sex, which correspond to the lower three chakras. A grounded consciousness in relation to money, food and sex (that fully relates to the issues of physical survival as a human being on planet Earth) is the foundation of happiness, but is by no means the peak. The consciousness must relate more fully in social love, self-love, and divine love, which correspond to the upper three chakras.

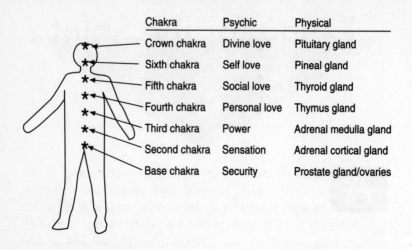

Chakra	Psychic	Physical
Crown chakra	Divine love	Pituitary gland
Sixth chakra	Self love	Pineal gland
Fifth chakra	Social love	Thyroid gland
Fourth chakra	Personal love	Thymus gland
Third chakra	Power	Adrenal medulla gland
Second chakra	Sensation	Adrenal cortical gland
Base chakra	Security	Prostate gland/ovaries

Additionally, the central chakra (the loving heart) must learn to respond without reservation. By reading this book you are working towards greater understanding of yourself in relation to food. This is an important step in your development.

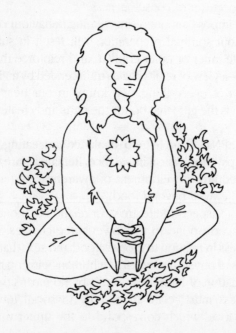

Eating for Happiness

If you base your happiness on indulging in a wide range of foods then your happiness may be even more short-lived than your body-mind. Unfortunately, our culture with its artificial environments and regimented lifestyles deprives many of us of the happiness of a peaceful and natural life. A persisting sense of deprivation may lead us to overindulge in food at every opportunity. As a result, we become flabbier, our skin deteriorates, and our physical attractiveness diminishes. This premature loss of physical beauty and aliveness compounds our sense of deprivation. Then we go to even greater extremes to satisfy our desires for stimulation. Many of us become enmeshed in this cycle of deprivation and indulgence, and see no way out.

Of course, there *is* a way out, but it is not advertised because some people make a lot of money from your unhappiness. I'll let you in on the secret: it is '10 Per Cent Conscious Debauchery'!

This 10 per cent of your total food intake can be *anything* you like! A marshmallow croissant, or a meat pie with sauce . . . anything. However, most importantly, you must indulge consciously, with full awareness. Try to be aware of the tastes and sensations and after-effects. In this way, with each indulgence you become more fully responsible for your indulgence. You have no guilt or regret, just awareness. For a few years after I began eating living foods I would occasionally indulge in a vegetable pie. Vegetable pie seemed a special food. When I decided to really taste every mouthful I realised how dry and tasteless it was; pastry seemed only a little better than cardboard. Now I am rarely impressed when I see a vegetable pie. Bananas and broccoli are much more attractive to me. It is often amazing how bad your favourite indulgence actually tastes when you eat it with intense awareness!

Now comes the crucial part. You have finished your 10 Per Cent Conscious Debauchery and you will probably say to yourself, 'Well, I've blown it now! I may as well forget about eating responsibly.' *No!* After your 10 Per Cent Conscious Debauchery you return to 90 Per Cent Purity without regrets, guilt, despair or deprivation. You simply return to 90 Per Cent Purity knowing that your time for responsible indulgence will come again!

Happiness comes out of freedom and caring. The CaPNaK Chart is not a rigid system; there is no fixed path for your wanderings around the chart. In fact, it is best if your path has a measure of chaotic unpredictability in which each day's eating is unique and unrepeated. However, this unpredictability must not be at the expense of your care for and responsiveness to the conditions of your body-mind.

The most common cause of nutritionally based unhappiness is a condition known as hypoglycaemia, or low blood-sugar level. When your blood-sugar level is low, your brain is deprived of its energy, and you feel grumpy, unhappy or irritable. You may also lose clarity, slur your speech, or begin to tremble. With a stable higher-blood-sugar level, you have a head-start on happiness.

You can stabilise your blood-sugar at a medium level by eating whole grains. The stomach has to work very hard to convert the big carbohydrate molecules into sugars. This is a slow process, so the blood-sugar never quite reaches high–energy levels. It is like putting ordinary petrol into a Formula One car—you become a plodder.

On the other hand, refined free sugars and stimulants boost the blood-sugar level too high too quickly. The body-mind reacts by releasing insulin to reduce the blood-sugar level. These sources of sugar are not in their natural form (that is, not integrated in living systems, as in fruit), and the naturally thinking body-mind reacts as if a large amount of fruit has been eaten and it releases too much insulin into the bloodstream. The insulin results in sugar being stored in the liver, leaving a low blood-sugar level. This perpetuates the craving for more sugar and stimulants.

Escaping the hypoglycaemic vicious circle is easy. Just eat more fruit. No, more fruit than that! Much more than that! Try about ten to fifteen pieces every day. Fruit is the high-octane fuel of the body-mind. The stomach takes control of the speed of release of sugar from the fruit's membranes to the duodenum, and hence to the bloodstream.

Fruit juice and dried fruit contain a high proportion of free sugars. To avoid destabilising your blood-sugar level, minimise the amount you consume of dried fruit and fruit juice.

You must learn to distinguish between your symptoms of low sodium and of low blood-sugar. These conditions are similar because they both create an energy low. See page 19 for the symptoms of underdose of sodium. Develop awareness of your blood-sugar level, and then consciously keep it high.

Graze on fruit whenever you feel yourself getting any low blood-sugar symptoms. Take fruit with you wherever you go, so that you always have the choice of body-mind happiness. When the living energy of fruit has washed away your toxic accumulations, every cell of your body-mind will sing with happiness.

Eating for Pleasure

Have you ever tried strawberries with avocado? How about cashews with baby bok choy, or whole canta- loupe followed by a banana. How about eating a peach or orange without chewing—just let the flesh slowly dissolve in your mouth. Try taking fifteen minutes to eat a banana.

Are you shocked by the intensity of the tastes? Eating slowly with awareness of every sensation can transform routine eating into paradisaical pleasure.

We are conditioned to believe that we must limit our experience of eating pleasure because it is fattening, expensive or unhealthy. True enough if it is a T-bone steak or black forest cake, but when it is unmutilated fruit and vegetables there are no limits. You can fill yourself up to the back of your throat with impunity, provided you wait until your stomach is empty before eating again. In fact, this conditioned limitation on how much you eat is one of the big hurdles to get over when you first start eating symbiotically. Beginners often do not eat enough, and consequently they lose too much weight, and then give up.

We all enjoy a social meal. Chatting and chewing is a valuable channel of communication, and symbiotic eaters should make every effort to stay at the table. If you want to avoid conflict, persistently steer the conversation away from your way of eating. Many people find health consciousness very confronting. Teach subtly through example.

If you are eating with people who appreciate fruit, then passing slices of fruit can become a bonding ritual. Oranges are already segmented for sharing. They are the symbiotic fruit of social beings.

At restaurants, you can base a healthy meal on appetisers, fruit and green salads. Eat the fruit salad first for correct food combining. Take a herbal tea bag, and order a cup of hot water. Ask for soup without bread, curry without rice, or baked vegetables without meat. Order an exotic fruit-juice mixture. Be creative. I am looking forward to the day when there are live-food restaurants, where every meal on the menu consists of living, unmutilated food.

You can hold a live-food banquet. I have attended wonderful banquets where the live food was not only delicious, but also presented in stunning colourful and sculptural dishes. See the recipes on pages 151–9 for a guide.

You can buy or grow a wide variety, including unusual greens: beet greens, dock, endive, turnip greens. You can experience the pleasure of wandering through a vegetable garden, picking leaves and piling them up as a leaf sandwich. You can make many exquisite, tangy combinations. Some fruit tree and vine leaves are also edible, but it is not advisable to eat leaves at random from your garden without checking that it is safe to do so.

I find the greatest pleasure in the simplicity of a banana dipped in carob powder, or mixing guacomale in my mouth by alternate bites on an avocado, tomato, and a clove of garlic. For sweets I like to suck some cinnamon bark, or mix one part carob powder with two parts unhulled tahini (from sesame seeds) as a chocolate substitute.

A scientist studying nutrition in monkeys (Milton 1993) put them on a diet of high-fibre, complex-carbohydrate foods. The monkeys were so displeased with eating mostly complex carbohydrates that they began to throw their food at the scientist! In the wild they only eat complex carbohydrates when there is no fruit. We primates find much more pleasure in the sweetness of fruit. However, complex carbohydrates, such as thin slices of sweet potato or pumpkin, are useful as a base for spreads such as avocado or tahini and/or salad.

Your transition to symbiotic eating may be helped by preparing living foods to look like your favourite mutilated foods of the past. Alternatively, completely let go of your memories of dead meals, and unequivocally embrace a symbiotic lifestyle. Just learn to fully appreciate what you are eating in each moment. If you are a good cook and enjoy mutilating foods, you may feel that a raw food lifestyle threatens your identity. Of course, you are absolutely correct, but what a wonderful opportunity to dissolve your identity in carrot juice and become enlivened! Think of the vast creative potential of preparing living foods in previously unheard-of ways; not to mention the healing forces you will unleash on your family and friends.

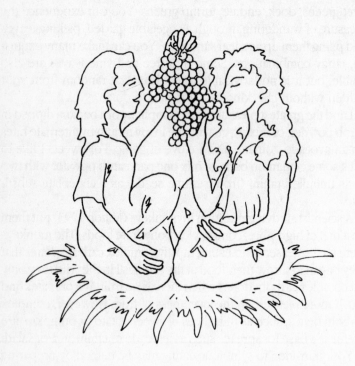

Eating for Cravings

Food cravings are the innate wisdom of your body-mind speaking to you; acknowledge and attend to them. Find a food that satisfies your craving. If a craving persists, then try to satisfy the craving by eating foods that you do not usually eat.

Pay attention to the taste. If the food tastes good to you, eat it, and observe the results. Remember the results. Learn. Craving indicates a nutritional deficiency. Discover what it is in a food that satisfies your craving. If necessary, find a healthier replacement, make affirmations, and integrate that replacement into your daily eating behaviour. Understand why you prefer certain foods to others. Go through the whole process again next time you have a craving. Refinement of your eating behaviour is progressive.

Sometimes I have a craving that I am not familiar with. In that case, I find it useful to tune in to the right food by holding various fruits and vegetables one at a time. I feel the reaction of my body-mind to each food as I hold them. Then I eat the food to which I feel the strongest attraction, usually with satisfying results.

Two familiar cravings are for sweet or savoury foods. After eating sweet foods such as fruit, we usually have a craving for savoury foods, and vice versa. You can understand this from the sodium-potassium balance on the CaPNaK Chart. Savoury foods are higher in sodium, and sweet foods lower, and therefore usually have a potassium-residue.

You can often understand cravings using the CaPNaK Chart. Many cravings are the result of an imbalance of the four primary minerals displayed on the chart. If your body-mind displays any of the symptoms of deficiency or overdose described earlier, then you can select an appropriate rebalancing food from the chart. The principle of replacing unhealthy foods with healthier foods is very important here.

I developed an occasional craving for potato crisps. Since there was not much else in those little plastic bags, I guessed it was the salt I was craving. After studying the sodium-residue end of the CaPNaK Chart, I decided that the healthiest source of sodium was green-leaf vegetables. When I increased my consumption of greens my craving for crisps reduced dramatically. In general, the need for artificial sources of salt is just a sign that the person is not eating enough greens—Macrobiotic and Asian-food eaters please note.

Eating for Addictions

Sugar is probably the most common addictive substance. It is hidden in many foods, or bravely displayed in the middle of the dining table. Every generation has to be informed about the many problems associated with sugar. Extracted simple carbohydrates (sugars) have many negative effects, such as those listed by Pritikin and McGrady (1973):

- increasing hunger unnecessarily
- stimulating insulin and fat production
- increasing blood triglycerides (fat)
- increasing blood cholesterol
- increasing uric acid in the blood
- promoting tooth decay.

Cigarettes, alcohol, coffee, tea and sweets all have a common addictive result: they all give a blood-sugar high. Alcohol and sweets give a direct blood-sugar high by supplying simple free carbohydrates, which the duodenum quickly injects into the bloodstream. Cigarettes, coffee and tea provide a blood-sugar high by stimulating the release of glucose from the liver by the action of nicotine and caffeine. Then, of course, there is chocolate, which provides blood-sugar both ways by directly supplying sugar and by stimulating release of sugar from the liver.

The blood-sugar high is a very pleasant state of contentment, and is a significant part of what the addict craves. The addictive components of tea, coffee, chocolate and cocoa are all chemically related to 'speed' (amphetamine).

You can circumvent the vicious circle of highs and lows in blood-sugar by eating fruit. Frequent eating of fruit (every hour or so) provides a very pleasant, stable high blood-sugar level. The blood-sugar level never drops, so the part of the addiction that is based on boosting blood-sugar levels disappears. It is then a lot easier to drop the unhealthy habits. First make fruit your positive addiction before you tackle your negative addictions.

On the other hand, if you smoke or drink regularly it is unwise to eat very low quantities of animal foods over many weeks, as the destruction of B vitamins alone can turn a smoking vegetarian into a 'vegetable'.

Broccoli is an antidote for the occasional hangover because of its high vitamin B content; it is also a good source for replenishing the minerals that you lose in urine after drinking alcohol. Caffeine also tricks the kidneys into pumping out essential vitamin and mineral reserves.

You also lose vitamin C if you smoke: each cigarette destroys about 25 mg. Smokers can reduce their chances of lung, throat and mouth cancers by eating lots of green-leaf vegetables. However, you must circumvent any routine substance-addiction, such as to alcohol or nicotine, before your symbiotic way of eating becomes too predominant. Simply begin by substituting healthier replacements for the addictive substances. Try to find food replacements that create a similar satisfaction of your needs. You may find it easier if you allow yourself to indulge in your addiction on particular days and times, and then gradually make those times further apart.

When I started eating symbiotically, I still smoked an occasional cigarette. I gradually weaned myself of my addiction by first using a filter whenever I smoked. Then I started mixing more and more coltsfoot tea (raspberry leaves are also good) with the tobacco, until finally I was smoking pure coltsfoot tea. Coltsfoot tea is not chemically addictive, so all I had to break then was the social and behavioural habit of smoking. From then on, every time I felt like a smoke I gave myself pain by wrapping my knuckles on the edge of a table! Soon I was associating smoking with pain—which is how it should be, considering the damage smoking does to your body-mind.

Eating for Travelling

Symbiotics should carry some fruit and green-leaf vegetables wherever they go. Until civilisation becomes supportive of eating unmutilated (uncooked) food, it will be difficult to buy fruit and greens in many places. A Symbiotic needs fast food just like anyone else in a modern lifestyle. However, there are few fast-unmutilated-food bars around, let alone live-food restaurants!

You'll feel better when flying if you steer clear of heavy meals, especially on long flights. Most airlines offer a variety of meals you can request in advance, including a fresh fruit platter. Take in plenty of non-alcoholic fluids and juicy foods to avoid being dehydrated by the plane's thirsty airconditioning system. Dehydration is a major cause of jetlag.

In normal circumstances, you do not need to drink anything when you eat living fruit and vegetables. Just eat fruit when you are thirsty, rather than dilute your digestion with water. When you carry fruit you need not carry a water bottle, and you have less likelihood of catching waterborne infections.

If you are travelling in places where hygiene or water is suspect, then you must peel your fruit. Alternatively, you can disinfect fruit by soaking it for twenty minutes in water containing six drops of Lugol's iodine solution in each litre (you can buy this solution from a chemist).

In such places, you must also eat mutilated vegetables, preferably boiled, but stir fried is also an option. Boiled spinach is often available, or you can order stir-fried vegetables at a Chinese restaurant. However, for your calcium needs eat at least 750 g (weight before mutilation) of greens every day (more for some women and older men; see Eating for Bone and Soft Tissue Health). If you eat less than this amount, then it is advisable to add the missing calcium with supplements, or by eating yogurt, real icecream, cheese, etc. Experiment to find out which dairy product provokes the least mucus in your throat.

If you catch the dreaded 'Delhi belly' or 'Montezuma's revenge', then match the liquidity of your food intake to that of your diarrhoea. Drink fruit and vegetable juice, with electrolyte replacement powder added, if available. Otherwise, add ½ tsp salt and 4 heaped tsp sugar to 1 litre water. Electrolyte powder provides sodium and potassium in the balanced ratio. The high potassium-residue of bananas will slow the bowels down and reduce the diarrhoea. Citrus fruits may help to kill the unwelcome bacteria by increasing the acidity of the upper digestive tract. Citric acid from fruit may also provide energy directly to your cells.

In places where ignorant or unscrupulous farmers may not have held fruit for a prescribed time after spraying, peel your fruit and vegetables. If no fruit is available, then potato or rice chewed thoroughly are the healthiest energy-food options. However, be sure to balance their acidity with some of the alkaline foods shown on the CaPNaK Chart. Carry some nuts or seeds, if you can buy them clean or in their shells.

If vegetables are unavailable or you feel the symptoms of being very low in sodium (such as feeling energetically drained, or having a weak digestion), you may need a quick fix. In such circumstances you can survive by eating some salt, or a salty snack such as potato crisps, until you obtain some green-leaf vegetables.

Recently, I worked in Tokyo as an electrical engineer. Rather than living in a little concrete room, I took my tent and found an overgrown area in the suburbs, on which there had once been a Zen school. I pitched my tent in the middle of a thicket, and lived there for many months. I commuted into central Tokyo for work, and wrote much of this book in the tent in my spare time. Being a live-food eater made camping very easy, since I had no need for water (I used bathroom facilities at a local shopping complex), fire or utensils. I enjoyed living in more extensive gardens than anyone else in Tokyo, besides the Emperor of course!

Eating for Sunshine

Sunshine is food-energy. The organised photons from the sun take food-energy to life. In scientific and meta-phorical terms, the biosphere is a dissipative structure swimming in the sun's river of light.

Humans and our primate ancestors wandered naked in the dappled sunlight of African jungles for millions of years. Our skin has evolved to accept plenty of sunlight, provided it is well nourished by the bloodstream. Furthermore, the body-mind needs sunlight. A well-known benefit of sunlight is that the ultraviolet light converts cholesterol to vitamin D. That cholesterol might otherwise be building up in the arteries! Instead, the vitamin D produced assists calcium absorption!

The increasing incidence of skin cancer and the destruction of the ozone layer are both now contributing to an increasing fear of sunshine. However, it is rarely mentioned that an important co-factor for skin cancer is the poor nutrition of the population.

For many people, the blood supply to the skin is obstructed by fat and cholesterol. Toxins are excreted through the skin, and some mutilated food components clog the oil glands. The blood flow becomes blocked, and adequate oxygen and nutrients cannot reach the skin (Horne 1985). If the blood flow is clear, damage done by solar radiation is much more easily repaired.

If adequate quantities of green-leaf vegetables are eaten, then the skin will contain large amounts of beta-carotene. Beta-carotene is an anti-cancer nutrient, which gives white skin a golden hue and protects it from sunlight, but it has the same protective effect whatever the colour of your skin. White skin has evolved in cold climates to reflect escaping heat back inside the body-mind. The skin can handle much more sunlight when it is protected by beta-carotene.

Carrot juice is notorious for turning you so amber that people think you are jaundiced. I remember entering a doctor's surgery where the nurse backed away thinking I had hepatitis! If you wish to avoid such a reaction, do not drink more than one glass of carrot juice a day.

Broccoli and many other greens are good sources of beta-carotene too. If your skin becomes too amber, then the antidote is half an hour of sunshine. Half an hour of sunshine every day is beneficial to well-nourished skin. However, we have not evolved to handle ozone holes, and let us make sure we don't have to! If an ozone hole is present, stay out of the sun between 10 a.m. and 2 p.m. (3 p.m. daylight saving time).

To keep cool in the sun see Eating for Cooling.

Eating for Beauty

Beauty is skin deep. There are few things so aesthetically pleasing as radiantly clear, smooth, silky skin. When you see such a person ask them if they eat much fruit. It is very likely you will get a yes. It is no secret that most of the beautiful people we see in film and print eat large amounts of raw food.

The balanced state of the body-mind is another, more subtle, source of beauty, a calm vitality that you can more easily achieve by eating living foods and by using mineral balancing as shown in the CaPNaK Chart. This provides a tranquil basis for enjoying life.

A major step towards beauty is to go within yourself and clarify the main disturbances of your body-mind. With persistence you will attain enough peace to begin bringing about deep changes in your lifestyle and behaviour. It is only then that you will be ready to improve your eating. First, you must drop destabilising stimulants (coffee, etc.) by replacing them with nature's natural stimulant: fruit.

You will then be moving towards low-fat and low-cholesterol eating, which will clear the blood supply to your skin. You will have less oil coming out of your pores. Providing you do not eat too much acid food (see the CaPNaK Chart), any acne will clear up in a few months. Beware of removing natural oils from the skin with soap and hot water. Warm water is enough to clean your skin without stripping off the protective natural oils, unless you are in a particularly dirty environment. If you insist on putting a skin cream on your face, use a thick cream. A thin cream or moisturiser is more likely to strip away your skin's natural oils. If you leave your natural oils intact, then in a matter of months your skin will be clear.

The most shapely, athletic, physically beautiful people I know all have one habit in common: they eat large quantities of raw vegetables. The minerals, amino acids, vitamins, and activated enzymes in living vegetables build tissue and bone into fabulous body-minds (see Eating for Bones and Soft Tissue Health, and Eating for Body Fluids Health). A friend of mine often used the terms 'meat-eater's butt' and 'rice chest' to describe some less-inspiring body shapes. Prematurely grey hair may be partly the result of a deficiency of PABA, a vitamin involved in hair pigmentation, skin health, and other processes. This is another nutrient supplied by green-leaf vegetables.

Your eyes are the jewels of your face. One particularly obvious signal of mineral balance occurs in the areas under your eyes. If you have dark areas under your eyes this is a sign you have been eating too much potassium-residue foods or not enough sodium-residue foods. Conversely, if there is an excess of extracellular fluid in your body-mind, then the fluid fills this space under your eyes, giving you the 'bags under your eyes' look. This is usually a result of eating too much sodium-residue or not enough potassium-residue foods. Adjust your sodium–potassium balance by consulting the CaPNaK Chart.

When you eat too much phosphorus-residue foods or not enough calcium-residue foods, dark scaly patches may form on your lips. These patches give your lips a rough and colourless texture. As you alkalise your body-mind with calcium-residue living foods your lips will become softer and redder.

The most detrimental factor to preserving physical beauty is smoking. Besides turning the body-mind into an acridly stinking waste dump, smoking replaces the oxygen in the blood with carbon monoxide. All the cells in the body-mind then become starved of oxygen and begin to shrivel up and malfunction. This is particularly noticeable with the skin. Smokers usually have pale chalky skin that starts to wrinkle up in their late twenties, at least ten years before its time. For information see Eating for Addictions.

It saddens me to see so much potential human beauty destroyed by ignorant choices. Beauty is yours to discover and choose, or you are responsible for its destruction. Find peace within, and then your steps towards beauty will be easy.

Eating for Elegance

Every year in midsummer on the north-east coast of Australia thousands of people become intoxicated with mango madness. They drive about for hours with glazed eyes in search of mango trees, and then arrive home with their cars full of their golden treasure trove. Frantic neighbours come running, throwing money, hoping to receive a share of the harvest Then the tragedy begins. Otherwise elegant people plunge their teeth into their mangoes, and immediately find their hands, face and clothes covered with sticky golden juice. You can avoid this undignified behaviour, by learning how to eat a mango without spilling a single drop:

1 Hold the lower end of the mango vertically in one hand, with the stalk-end uppermost.

2 With the other hand, carefully peel strips of skin vertically downwards, similarly to a banana, from the top end to two-thirds down the length of the mango.

3 Gently eat the mango from the top down, being careful to give a final suck to remove superfluous juice each time you tear the flesh away with your teeth.

4 When you have eaten the exposed flesh, place the exposed end of the seed in your mouth; and then, while withdrawing the mango from your mouth, scrape the seed clean with your teeth.

5 Repeat step 4 until that end of the seed is clean and free of juice; then take hold of the seed with your free hand, and turn the mango upside down.

6 Holding the mango by the seed, carefully peel the skin off the end of the mango. Eat the remainder of the mango according to step 3.

7 Throw the mango seed in any place you would like to see a mango tree grow. There can never be enough mango trees!

If you follow these instructions carefully, you will be counted among the elegant elite of mango munchers. Use similar eating techniques for many other fruits so that your cutlery and crockery can join the stove at the garbage dump. Now you can turn the kitchen into that spare bedroom you always wanted!

There are many fruits that you don't need to peel at all. These include kiwi fruit (just rub the hairs off and bite in!) passionfruit (the skin is tasty, and chewy, when combined with the juice and seed). The CaPNaK Chart shows passionfruit as being acid. Maybe, if the skin had been included in the analysis, the result for passionfruit would have been less acid.

My home is a greenhouse grotto with a translucent roof, allowing many plants to grow inside. I call it an 'ecome' because it is environmentally very friendly, and has a minimum of wood and other materials in its construction. Flowers, ferns and vegetables grow on the sloping walls, and vines cross the trellis ceiling. One of these is a prolific passionfruit vine, and almost every morning I find a delicious passionfruit that has fallen onto my grass carpet.

Eating for Peace

Most of us long for a peaceful life in which we can pursue creative or productive work. However, if the neighbours take over our backyard, there is every chance of conflict. We organise socially and economically to control and regulate such conflicts of needs. Nevertheless, the global organisation necessary to assure international peace is still in the making.

We can encourage fairer use of agricultural land by choosing foods that do not demand an unfair share of resources. Cattle farming requires a relatively large area of land per kilojoule of food produced. Populations go hungry as their farmlands grow cattle feed for richer nations. Half of the world's grain harvest is fed to livestock while 20 million people die every year from malnutrition and starvation (EarthSave 1992). There is no other single food that produces so much suffering, starvation, and sickness, both in the producing and the consuming nations as does beef.

Meat consumption is also a disruptive force in our personal experience of inner peace. The high sodium, phosphorus and protein levels and the hormones in meat form a chemical cocktail leading to anxiety and aggression. Add to this the blood-sugar fluctuations created by sugar and other stimulants, and we have a menu for escalating inner and outer conflict. When peace finally comes it is in the form of tranquillisers.

If we replace cattle farming with the growing of fruit it will lead to a fairer, more local distribution of this less transportable food. Through the consumption of fruit it will lead to the experience of inner peace among ever-widening circles of people.

We need not retreat to the forest to live in peace; there is great potential for us to live more peacefully in cities, especially if we reduce, and respond more effectively to, the physiological and social sources of stress. We must nurture the rest-and-digest response daily, by taking time for meditative contemplation. No one needs the addition of inner stress created by indigestion and imbalanced eating. The CaPNaK Chart addresses this question of imbalance.

Two peaceful CaPNaK forces are available: potassium-residue for passivity; calcium-residue for tranquillity. These peaceful forces are combined in foods in the yin–alkaline quadrant. It is worth noting that meats are in the diametrically opposite quadrant of the CaPNaK Chart. You can create more passive tranquillity in your life by eating more yin–alkaline foods.

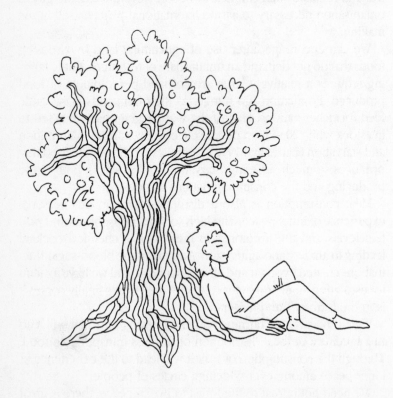

Eating for Satisfaction

You will sometimes feel a gnawing need for something filling. You may then move into a state of consciousness called 'the unbearable lightness of being a Symbiotic'. Of course, this is a state of imbalance. It can be cured by eating phosphorus-residue foods such as bananas, avocados or nuts. Two or three bananas are usually enough to banish that empty feeling. Eat too many, and you may come in for a crash landing.

You can find other food options that satisfy this craving in the phosphorus-residue half (the bottom half) of the CaPNaK Chart. See Eating for Cravings for more information.

Some people complain that it would be boring to eat mostly fruit. These people should look in a good fruit shop and see the incredible range of fruits that nature provides. Look beyond the apples and oranges at the mangoes, avocados, persimmons, durians and sapotes! And what is in the shop is only a tiny fraction of what you can grow.

An incredible range of vegetables, herbs, nuts and seeds can be eaten raw. Stock up on a wide range so that you can combine them in interesting ways to satisfy your wants. Some unusual varieties are available.

Dissatisfaction with symbiotic eating cannot be fairly blamed on lack of variety. Cultural conditioning into our present 'culture of death' is the true basis of dissatisfaction. If we want a healthier life and planet, we have to accept the need to recondition ourselves into a 'culture of life'.

Fruit	Vegetables	Herbs	Nuts and seeds
blueberry	artichoke	chamomile	Brazil
cumquat	collard	coriander	cashew
fig	cress	dandelion	linseed
guava	endive	fennel	macadamia
loquat	kale	lemongrass	pecan
persimmon	kohlrabi	liquorice	pepita
pomegranate	okra	mace	pine nut
prickly pear	rutabaga	peppermint	pistachio
quince	turnip	saffron	sesame
tangelo	yam	turmeric	sunflower

Eating for Money

People often think that Symbiotic eating is too expensive. Sure, fruit is expensive, but so are cheese, meat, and other processed foods. If you add up your food bills, you will find that fruit-oriented eating will cost about the same as other eating styles. A bland and lifeless rice diet may be a little cheaper.

Next, add in the costs of energy for refrigeration, food mutilation and washing up. Include the environmental costs of packaging, processing, etc., and the cost of your future cardiovascular bypass operation and physiotherapy. Symbiotic eating comes out way ahead. Money does grow on trees after all!

Of course, if you have some space and time for a vegetable garden or some fruit trees, you can cut your food bill considerably. However, many of us have less time than money. If, for you, time is money, read Eating for Time.

An Institute of Health and Welfare study (1994) showed that poor eating habits cost Australians three billion dollars a year in health care. This takes no account of the social and commercial costs of illness. I think it would be a much higher figure if the full human potentials for health and longevity were recognised.

The direct cost of health-care service for diet-related diseases was estimated to be $1862 million in 1989–90. Indirect costs of illness and death to the economy was estimated to be $1418 million, resulting in a total of $3280 million in 1989–90 (Australian Institute of Health 1994, p. 55).

Eating for Time

I know that time is an illusion, but I wonder why it took me so long to find out? While I ponder the entropic implication of this neurologic irritation, time has been quietly eating itself somewhere deep inside my watch.

Time just gets hungrier when you fill it with shopping, food preparation and washing-up. How many hours a week do people spend rattling pots and pans, and shuttling between the butcher, baker, and milk bar? This is possibly the greatest waste of human resources on the planet; regardless of the sick days, and hours of low energy, produced by eating mutilated food.

Life is easier when you shop only at the greengrocer's. Life is a dream when food preparation means rearranging the fruit bowl. Life is a laugh when washing-up becomes wiping your hands and licking your lips.

A fruit-eater has such an easy time digesting that at least one hour's less sleep is required. Also, with a quick bite (bite quickly, but chew slowly) on an apple or broccoli, you can blend the actual eating with other activities and work. If you cannot snack on fruit while you are working, then fill up on fruit during tea breaks. You will have no problem eating three pieces of fruit in ten minutes, if necessary.

Consequently, you can easily release an extra four or five hours per day for creative, productive and caring activities or contemplation—and have the stable high blood-sugar necessary to use that time well! Can you imagine a whole civilisation with such an increase of human capacity? Frankly, I cannot, because it would be absolutely awesome.

Eating for Sleep

Most of us spend between six and nine hours each day sleeping, so it is worth carefully considering how eating can aid sleeping.

While you sleep, your body-mind is busy eliminating. You are preparing for the next day. The more you eat, the more you have to eliminate, and the more sleep you will need. If you combine your foods badly, then the elimination process will take longer, and you will need more sleep.

Some people have trouble sleeping because they have to get up to urinate during the night. If you eat symbiotic food, you get large amounts of water in the food. The unmutilated food has not been dried by heating, and it provides the body-mind with its full requirements of water. Drinking extra beverages adds unnecessary extra water for a Symbiotic. If you eat or drink within two or three hours of your bedtime you load up your bladder, and this will interrupt your sleep.

Do you wake up feeling drained and weak? You may be sleeping in a bed that is too hot. If your bed is too hot, you lose too much sodium and water in perspiration, and you wake up with symptoms of potassium overdose (see page 19). Before I understood CaPNaK balancing I often had mouth ulcers, and thought I had inherited a predisposition from my mother. However, my mouth ulcers ceased when I began to pay more attention to reducing the number of blankets on my bed! When you overheat in bed you tend to breathe through your mouth. Your body is cooled by evaporation as the air passes over your mouth's mucous membranes. Ulcers tend to form in the dried mucous membranes. Overheating in bed inhibits REM (rapid eye movement or dreaming state) sleep, and leaves you with a hangover in the morning. Use fewer blankets, and use doonas only in particularly cold climates.

If I dine out and eat a meal based on grain, then I usually wake up very early the next morning. This happens despite my need for extended elimination. It is probably due to the sudden overdose of phosphates from the grain, which create an acidic condition. Insomnia is a symptom of acidosis (see page 19). The antidote is calcium-rich foods, such as green-leaf vegetables. I recommend eating plenty of broccoli, as soon as possible after eating grain, to re-alkalize your body-mind.

If you suffer from insomnia, a few simple behavioural changes may improve your sleep. When you wake up, get out of bed immediately, and don't take a nap during the day; this ensures that you will need to sleep when you go to bed at night. If you eat or drink stimulants, don't do so after midday. Replace stimulants with nature's stimulant: fruit.

Eating for Work

I n the bad old days, before I started eating symbiotically, I had problems with running out of energy in the afternoon. I began keeping a packet of barley sugar on my desk, and eating one every fifteen minutes to boost my blood-sugar level. However, I could feel those nutritionally empty kilojoules draining my health away.

You can only properly satisfy your natural, primate craving for sweetness by a constant supply of blood-sugar (see Eating for the Past). The best source of stable, high blood-sugar is from the continuous breakdown of fruit in your digestive tract. The idea is to eat so much fruit that your whole abdomen is full of fruit in various stages of digestion. Grazing is the key; don't wait for mealtimes, eat whenever you feel the urge.

Nowadays, I keep the bottom drawer of my filing cabinet at work stocked with fruit, green-leaf vegetables, and unhulled tahini or nuts. While reading, writing, telephoning, computing, or during discussions, I can reach down and grab a banana. There is no separation; working and eating are one. It is very unlikely that you will attract condemnation unless you make a big deal out of it. After all, people have been discreetly snacking at their desks since paperwork began.

If your job is more physically oriented, and not desk-bound, then you may have to restrict your eating to breaks. Then you must load up with enough fruit to avoid hunger pangs until the next break. Three pieces of fruit should be sufficient for two hours. It is a good idea to save the 'fast fruits' such as bananas and apples for the moments when you need a quick snack. Eat the messier fruit like oranges during breaks. Take a short walk out of the office if you want to avoid the smell of oranges permeating the office.

Save your salad for the lunch break when you have more time to eat. Broccoli rolled in lettuce leaves, or an alkaline salad such as the lunch salad given in the recipes in Part 2, is a natural tranquilliser to counteract stress. If you need some yang energy to boost your strength and motivation, munch on some celery or other food at the sodium-residue side of the CaPNaK Chart. You will feel the effects beginning after about 15–30 minutes. The more physical your work is, the more fat and sodium you will need; see Eating for Action, and Eating for Thought.

Walk to the greengrocer's at lunchtime to replenish your filing cabinet, and get some exercise. If you are invited to an office party, take a few pieces of fruit in your briefcase, and also eat plenty of salad. If you drink alcohol, eat lots of broccoli afterwards to boost your vitamin B. If you find yourself getting too angry or aggressive towards your colleagues, you can pacify yourself with yin foods such as bananas, apricots, dates or okra. Again you will feel the effects beginning after 15–30 minutes.

If you work indoors, try to get a little sunshine on your skin every day, to produce sufficient vitamin D. A deficiency of sunshine will also make you feel depressed. I recommend that you buy a negative-ion generator to freshen up the air around your desk, especially if there is a lot of electronic equipment (or smoke) in your office.

I do not advise eating fruit in the middle of a formal meeting! Keep some dried fruit handy for such occasions. Ask your boss to buy a juicer for the tea-room.

Eating for Action

How you eat for action depends on the action you are doing. Do you need aerobic energy or anaerobic strength?

Aerobic energy requires a free-flowing bloodstream to supply copious quantities of oxygen and glucose to the muscles. For this, you need lots of fruit and a minimum of fat, preferably from nuts and avocado. Fat makes your blood cells sticky and slows the flow. You also need to eat high-sodium-residue green-leaf vegetables such as celery to supply sodium to keep you cool.

Anaerobic strength is not the exclusive domain of hulks. Champion weightlifter Wiley Brooks of Venice, California, is 183 cm tall and weighs 61 kg, but has lifted 424 kg. He eats only raw fruit and fruit juice. During anaerobic exercise your muscles burn more fat and less carbohydrate. So it makes sense to prepare for anaerobic exercise by eating more fats from avocados and nuts. For heavy anaerobic work even two or three large avocados a day would be OK. Do not continue a high fat intake for an extended period.

Holistic physical health cannot result only from the way you eat. Exercise is another important factor. If you think of exercise as a chore or unproductive drain on your energy, try to create your exercise through your usual daily activities. Walking is an excellent form of exercise. Walk to the shops or railway station instead of driving. Take a stroll in a park or mall during lunchtime, or along a beach or in a forest at the weekend. When you stretch in the morning or at your desk, try doing some real yoga assanas instead. An assana is a pose or stretch you do with awareness of your body-mind and breathing. Just simply touching your toes can be done as an assana. Go to a yoga class to learn how to develop and expand your awareness of your body-mind. You don't have to be a sportsperson to get enough exercise.

Eating for Sport

Some people believe that consumption of animal products is essential for strength, endurance and general health. There are many examples of vegan and vegetarian athletes—for example, Dave Scott, six-time winner of the Ironman Triathlon; Sixto Linanes, holder of world records in twenty-four-hour triathlons, etc.

Dehydration is the biggest enemy of athletes. The loss of 1 litre of body water results in a 15 per cent drop in physical power output (Haas 1983). Raw fruit and vegetables are a good source of mineralised water. Drink water, or eat juicy fruit, before, during and after a sports event. Don't wait for a thirst before you drink. Chilled liquids are absorbed faster into your blood.

Low blood-sugar, called 'bonking' by athletes (which proves some don't get enough leisure time), results in the shakes, tiredness and incoherent thinking. Your aim should be to prevent, not relieve, bonking by eating fruit in sufficient quantities before the event. Fruit juices should be avoided because they destabilise blood-sugar levels.

Salt tablets require water to be diverted to your stomach, resulting in internal dehydration. This occurs to a lesser extent with sodium-residue juices and foods. Sports drinks reach your blood much more slowly than water, and tend to be too concentrated and thus draw water out of your muscles. Protein foods also promote dehydration (Haas 1983).

When an athlete 'hits the wall', the muscles run out of glycogen. (The muscles need glycogen as their fuel, so without it you feel like you are trying to walk through a wall.) Fruit replenishes the muscles' stores of glycogen. Fasting robs athletes of endurance by depleting muscle tissue, glycogen, vitamins and minerals.

Sports injuries heal more quickly with low-fat food, particularly because of the reduction of free-radical damage (see Eating for Longevity). Antioxidant foods also speed healing.

Speed up your metabolism to get your body-mind operating faster. I have discussed how to do this in Eating for Weight Loss. To increase muscle mass, do exercise such as weight training, and eat more total kilojoules rather than increasing protein intake.

Jogging, skiing, swimming and aerobic dancing are endurance sports requiring aerobic metabolism. Running, swimming, cycling and martial arts also demand some anaerobic activity.

Here is some specific advice for particular types of sports.

In the dietary suggestions below, one piece of fruit is taken as 150 g (e.g. a medium banana or medium orange). The quantities given are the maximum amounts that could be consumed by world-class athletes in rigorous training. Weekend athletes would not need nearly as much.

Basic Intake

Each day eat fruit to the equivalent of 1680 kilojoules (about 1 kg or 7 pieces) for each hour of your sport; *plus* up to 1 kg green leaf vegetables and up to 50 g nuts and seeds, daily; *plus* the following food in your sport category.

Category 1: Aerobic dancing, cycling, jogging, skiing, and swimming

These sports involve aerobic exercise, which occurs when the pulse exceeds 120 beats per minute. Eat low-fat, low-cholesterol, high-carbohydrate, high-enzyme food: 28 pieces of fruit (4 kg) a day, plus the Basic Intake.

Category 2: Baseball, basketball, boxing, football, karate, and soccer

Sports in this category require bursts of energy, which demand a higher kilojoule intake. Eat up to 49 pieces of fruit (7 kg) a day, plus the Basic Intake. You might need to use a blender to enable you to eat this much!

Category 3: Tennis

Eat 21 pieces of fruit (3 kg) a day, plus the Basic Intake.

Category 4: Weights

Largely anaerobic exercise; eat 42 pieces of fruit (6 kg) a day, plus the Basic Intake.

Category 5: Golf

Eat 14 pieces of fruit (2 kg) a day, plus the Basic Intake. Eat fruit during play to feed the brain with a high blood-sugar level.

After your sporting event eat the following uncooked meal: 150 g broccoli, 300 g peas, 7 pieces (1 kg) of fruit, and drink water, according to thirst, if necessary.

Some athletic sports, such as long-distance running, are in category 1, and others such as sprinting fall between categories 1 and 2.

Eating for Thought

A sincere seeker of truth once told me that the brain is merely an energy storage system, and does not form a basis for thinking processes. However true that may be for him, the rest of us suffer a high drain on our energy supply by the brain, especially during intense mental activity.

About 30 per cent of the total energy released from food is used in the brain. As distinct from the muscles, which burn both carbohydrate and fat, the brain burns only carbohydrate for energy. A stable, high blood-sugar level is important for sustained thinking, and fructose from fruit is an excellent source of blood-sugar.

So, if you have some intense mental work to do, keep a fruit bowl within arm's reach, and keep munching. If you want to turn up the intensity further, then try eating only the fruit shown in the acid area of the CaPNaK Chart. This will increase your level of anxiety, as noted in the symptoms of acidosis on page 19. Moderate anxiety can improve your performance.

The amino acid, phenylalanine, gives a brain boost and also suppresses the appetite. Apricot, bean sprout, broccoli, fig, kale, peanut, pea, potato, pumpkin and sesame seeds, spinach, and turnip green, are all good sources. This is particularly good if you want to lose weight, and think at the same time.

If you are an office worker, see Eating for Work for more information about excellent eating in the office.

It does not take too much deep thinking to see some of the connections between our eating choices and the overwhelming demands on the environment, the Earth's resources, and our health. With your thought processes in higher gear you will see even more clearly and assume increasing responsibility regarding human nutrition and our planetary emergency.

Eating for Emotions

A major and widespread cause of emotional instability is hypoglycaemia or low blood-sugar. The symptoms of hypoglycaemia include:

- brief periods of depression
- difficulty concentrating before lunch or dinner
- swings from very high to very low energy during a normal day
- frequent bouts of anxiety or nausea
- irritability and tension
- severe headaches, lightheadedness, or feeling faint if you haven't eaten for a while
- constantly hungry
- nervousness, or trouble sleeping
- cold, clammy skin.

Free sugars and stimulants contribute to this worldwide plague of hypoglycaemic mood swings. Humans consume free sugars and stimulants in massive quantities in soft drinks, coffee, tea and cigarettes. A first step towards emotional stability must include the replacement of free sugars and stimulants by the natural stimulation of fruit.

Mutilated food has a tremendously destabilising effect on blood-sugar levels. Fluctuation of your blood-sugar level from eating mutilated food can be ten times greater than is caused by live or enzyme-rich food (Santillo 1987). By eating live food, you experience a much steadier metabolic rate and emotional stability.

Once you have swept aside the irritabilities, anxieties and depressions of hypoglycaemia, then you can move into a more subtle awareness of, and influence over, your emotional states. Using the CaPNaK Chart you can eat:

- calcium-residue foods for more sensitivity and calmness
- phosphorus-residue foods for more resilience and intensity
- sodium-residue foods for more activity and dominance
- potassium-residue foods for more passivity and gentleness.

Of course, food can only influence the emotional state; it cannot control it! For example, bananas cannot turn raving mania into gentle peacefulness, but they may bring a little passivity.

Everyone experiences emotional events in their lives. The distress and disturbance created by these events can play havoc with our intentions to eat well. Resolving emotional difficulties is an important part of maintaining health of the body-mind.

If you ignore your emotional response to an event, you must repress your feelings on some level of your body-mind. Eventually, repressed feelings bubble up, and you may lose control in ways not directly related to the original event, for example, you may go on a food binge. If you acknowledge your emotional reaction when it first occurs, you can spend some time fully experiencing and observing your emotions. When you have resolved the issues both internally and in relationships, your emotions dissipate. Then there will be no disruption to other aspects of your life, including your healthy eating.

Many people feel threatened by someone who does not conform to their idea of what is 'normal'. When you become a live-food eater, you may encounter family and peer-group pressure challenging your emotional wellbeing. Take care in discussing your new way of eating, because simple questions can turn into emotional attacks if your answers are naive or condescending. Many people respond emotionally to issues about food, and can easily feel offended when confronted by your new approach to your food. However, it is important to discuss your experiences with those who are genuinely interested: a small insight from such a discussion might have an enormous impact on such pople.

You will experience symptoms of withdrawal from your previous foods if you try to make the transition to living food too quickly. You may then experience frustration and stress, which can throw your body-mind off-balance. In Eating for the Evolution of Consciousness I introduced the idea of food chakras. Take another look at the foods associated with each food chakra. You can ease your transition to living foods by moving your eating habits month by month up the food chakras. The closer you already are to live-food eating, the faster your transition will be. If you have any physical or mental upsets as a result of your transition, then slow down your changes. Be patient: the physiological and mental conditioning of your old ways of living will eventually fall away, leaving you fully enlivened!

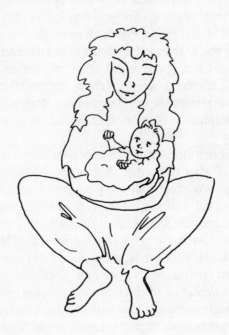

Eating for Personality

Have you ever considered eating your way to a different personality, or perhaps a more balanced personality? It is interesting to speculate about some apparent correlations between food and personality. More specifically, Carl Jung's four basic personality types have some correlations with the predominant states of the body-mind induced by the four CaPNaK minerals. These personality types are the thinker (or intellectual), the feeler (or performer), the intuitive (or entertainer), and the sensitive (or director) (Jung 1971). These personality types are related to each other diagrammatically as shown. Think of an individual personality as a single point in one of the quadrants of the diagram.

Intuitive—the entertainer (love)	Feeler— the performer (beauty)			Ca	Alkaline
		Na			K
Sensitive— the director (goodness)	Thinker— the intellectual (truth)	Yang			Yin
				P	Acid

Correspondence between Jung's personality types and the CaPNaK Chart.

Both left-hand quadrants are extroverted personalities; both right-hand quadrants are introverted personalities. Both upper quadrants are people-oriented personalities; both lower quadrants are task-oriented personalities. The spiritual orientation of each personality type is shown in parentheses.

133

The correspondence with the CaPNaK Chart is a direct mapping, as follows: the sodium–calcium-residue quadrant corresponds to the intuitive personality; the sodium–phosphorus-residue quadrant corresponds to the sensitive personality; the potassium–calcium-residue quadrant corresponds to the feeler personality; the potassium–phosphorus-residue quadrant corresponds to the thinker personality.

If there is any causal relationship between these personality types and the tendency to prefer particular mineral-residue foods, the relationship may operate both ways. The personality influences the food preference; the food preference influences the personality. In my experience, the CaPNaK system offers this potential for you to expand your personality development. It is a yoga of food.

Eating for Sex

Eating fruit is actually a very sexual activity—after all, you are in fact eating trees' genitals! Also many fruits have quite suggestive shapes, colours and textures; this makes sense, given their symbiotic need to attract primates and other fruit-eating species. Sharing a banana or a juicy peach with your lover can be a sensual experience to complement the joys of sex.

For millenia, people have sought secret aphrodisiacs from far-away lands, but some simple everyday foods can have profound effects on the libido. You may be feeling drained and weak but your lover is overwhelmed by desire—try chomping your way through a few sticks of celery or other high sodium-residue food. This will boost the volume of your extracellular fluid, including your blood volume, thus making available a little extra blood pressure for those dizzy heights of ecstasy. If your partner has a lower interest in sex, try slipping a bit of seaweed into the salad. The iodine present may stimulate the thyroid to promote the flow of hormones.

Certain 'precious bodily fluids' are more readily replaced when you eat avocados, pumpkin seeds (pepitas) and nuts. Pumpkin seeds are a particularly good source of zinc (6.6 mg/100 g), which is lost in semen. Green-leaf vegetables (0.7 mg/100 g) and mush-rooms (1.2 mg/100 g) are also good sources of zinc. Small doses of testosterone are reputed to wildly heighten the female libido. I'll leave it to your imagination to discover how natural emissions of traces of this hormone can be devoured!

Women who take birth-control pills containing oestrogen may gain some weight. You can reduce this problem by activating more lipolytic enzymes to burn fat by exercising a little more; for example, do a few laps around your mattress before you go to sleep. See also Eating for Weight Loss.

Excess body fat can upset the sex-hormone balance, and reduce sexual desire. Sexual activity can also be adversely affected by cardiovascular diseases.

Reduction or cessation of menstrual flow often accompanies fruit-oriented eating. This may not necessarily affect ovulation. It appears the menstrual process can occur with little loss of blood and it is more widely accepted, even among some conventional medical experts, that this reduction or cessation may be a sign of improved health (Horne 1985, p. 330). Some writers such as Horne have strongly argued that the primary function of menstruation is to expel wastes and detoxify the reproductive system; if the food eaten generates less wastes and toxins, as symbiotic eating undoubtedly does, then the menstrual flow can be significantly lighter without increasing any toxicity in the body-mind. Nevertheless, the current view of medical experts (such as Haas 1983) is that menstrual diminution is an abnormality induced by nutritional stress. Amenorrhea (irregular or missed menstrual periods) may occur if your body fat is below 15 per cent. This may be an adaptation to reduce the incidence of pregnancy in times of food shortage. In this case, the fruit-based diet may be an excellent substitute for contraception—just binge for ovulation? Some fruit-eaters induce nutritional stress by simply not eating enough. Remember: a fruit-oriented diet must include at least 2 kg fruit every day to provide sufficient kilojoules. An average-sized woman should manage to eat 2.5 kg fruit, an average-sized man 3 kg, in addition to the greens, seeds and nuts I recommend.

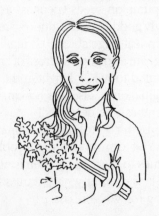

Eating for Children

We don't inherit the land from our ancestors, we borrow
it from our children—Pennsylvania Dutch saying

D on't wait until you are pregnant to be health conscious.
Eating healthily won't make you pregnant, but it will
help you grow a healthy baby. You can reduce the
chance of infertility and miscarriage by maintaining a vitalised and
detoxified body-mind. Miscarriage often occurs as a result of stress,
and food-stress from toxic, denatured foods should not be overlooked as a significant factor. Do not attempt a transition to a
living-food diet during pregnancy; during transition toxic wastes
stored in the mother's body will be released into the bloodstream,
and may affect the foetus.

Increased protein intake during pregnancy leads to increased
birth weights for infants only as long as protein does not exceed
25 per cent of the kilojoules eaten. Higher protein intake than that
leads to lower birth weights (Dunbar 1991). Green-leaf vegetables
are a good source of protein. For example, broccoli contains 27 per
cent protein by kilojoules. Try to satisfy any craving for protein by
first eating green-leaf vegetables.

During pregnancy your oestrogen and body fat levels will
increase. Your body needs some extra body fat, but don't overindulge. Just eat healthily to satisfy your hunger, and keep
exercising your body. You may not lose your extra fat as a result of
breastfeeding, but exercise will activate your lipolytic enzymes to
trim and tone up your body. Go for walks or bicycle rides with your
baby.

Mother's milk has a large amount of live enzymes and all of the
nutrients needed for the growth of your infant. Milk formulas lack

137

enzymes. The mortality rate of artificially-fed infants is about fifty times greater than among the breast-fed (Santillo 1987).

You will find human milk on the CaPNaK Chart near the green-leaf vegetables. Note that breast milk has less calcium- and sodium-residue than cow's milk; humans do not need to develop massive bones like cattle. Breast milk also contains about 6 per cent protein (by kilojoules), which is similar to fruit. A baby doubles its weight in six months on this amount of protein. Considering that adults have no such growth requirement, it is little wonder that they receive adequate protein by eating fruit, nuts and green-leaf vegetables!

Remember that pesticides used in agriculture are concentrated by the food chain from vegetables to animals. Beware of putting yourself at the end of the food chain:

• the amount of non-vegetarian mother's milk with significant levels of the pesticide DDT in America is 99 per cent
• the amount of vegetarian mother's milk with significant levels of DDT is 8 per cent (EarthSave Foundation 1992).

Excessive intake by pregnant women of any one food should be avoided, for example 2 litres a day of carrots or parsley for several days would be excessive.

As you wean your child, breast milk is best replaced by fruit and green-leaf vegetables. Children instinctively enjoy fruit. Every 100 mg of calcium they need can be supplied by a little more than 100 g of green-leaf vegetables. Include nuts only when the child is old enough to safely chew and digest them. Occasional sources of vitamin B_{12} in the diet are important for the development of a child's nervous system.

Some fruit-conscious mothers tell me that oranges can create problems for babies wearing nappies. Something in oranges that passes out in faeces and urine when retained by a nappy can burn the baby's bottom. Maybe someone will invent a symbiotic nappy made from banana leaves?

One of the few things that all humans have in common is eating. Eating is a good way to share time together, but why teach children, against their instincts, to eat a predetermined meal of mutilated food? Peace can reign in the family where each child learns self-regulated eating. When you eat together, provide nuts, seeds, herbs, spices, toppings, dressings and dips for each person to alter their fruit and vegetables according to their tastes. Ensure that there is a wide variety of fruits and vegetables available. Provide dried fruit if anyone has an unsatisfied sweet tooth.

To encourage children to eat intuitively, allow them to graze from bowls of fruit, green-leaf vegetables and nuts (for those old enough). The children then quickly gain mastery over their eating choices and do not get traumatised by the disempowerment and choicelessness of a family meal of deadened food. The brightness and joy of a child fed on living foods is a pleasure to see.

Store fruit in a prominent position to encourage all the family to eat it as a snack. Use fruit as a decoration in your house. Avoid eating overripe or underripe fruit; overripe fruit usually has a clear appearance inside, and begins to smell fermented.

Most schoolchildren lack food enzymes (Santillo 1987). This shortfall lays the foundation for allergies, obesity, constipation and fatigue; children who maintain high enzyme levels maintain high energy levels. Overfeeding your child, especially with heat-mutilated food, requires the digestive organs to secrete large amounts of enzymes daily. Over a period of time your child's enzyme-producing organs become exhausted, and immunity is weakened.

Avoid feeding your child too much calcium-residue food. While adequate calcium builds thick, strong bones, excessive calcium can stunt growth. Alkaline people tend to have shorter and stockier builds.

Eating for Getting High

A natural high is associated with the stable, high blood-sugar levels attained with fruit-eating. Many creatures in the wild get drunk when the wild fruits ferment, and their drunken feasts are a natural part of their life-cycles. At times, the Symbiotic may be slightly, and pleasantly, inebriated; especially when grapes and watermelons are in season.

An important psychoactive factor is the alkalinity of foods. A rapid alkalisation of the bloodstream can have a pleasant temporary effect: the body is filled with a feeling of deep relaxation, the mind becomes happy, tranquil and calm, the senses are hightened and brightened. Juice a large amount (up to 50 g) of parsley mixed in a cup of carrot juice (to reduce the acidity of carrot juice, stir the carrot pulp into the juice). Drink a litre or two of this elixir, then sit back, relax, and enjoy the experience. This must not be drunk by pregnant women, since large amounts of parsley can cause abortion.

Many psychoactive herbs and fungi can be eaten raw with varying degrees of legality and toxicity; for example, tobacco, hops, marijuana, opium, cocaine, and mushrooms. Plants have their own purposes in the evolution of their addictiveness; for example, they spread their seeds or get fertilised by attentive and addicted animals. You may dance with a plant, but watch who leads the dance. Treat this power of nature with respect so that it does not turn into a triple-headed dragon that haunts you with its fiery breath! In other words: beware of addiction. Unfortunately, we have lost our sacred rites in which drug-taking was constrained by rituals. Now we have discos and bars where constraint is supplanted by promotion, and transcendence is replaced by escapism. Use has become abuse: eating power-plants has been replaced by smoking, drinking or injecting them.

Eating for the Environment

Phosphorus poisoning is one of our all-round blind spots: both personal and planetary! We acidify our bodies with excessive phosphorus-residue foods. It is rather ironical that we are also acidifying our soils with phosphate fertiliser.

Acidic fertilisers become more and more necessary to leach the remaining trace minerals from our overworked soils. After a few decades our soil becomes deficient in some minerals, and cannot support a healthy crop. A solution is to put back into the soil the trace minerals that we have taken away in the harvest. We can do this by recycling organic matter as compost, and spreading finely-ground rock dust onto the soil. Organic farming depends on maintaining the micro-organisms in the soil. These break down trace rock minerals, and integrate them into protoplasm. The plants then feed on the protoplasm. This works best if you recycle organic waste that is not already mineral deficient. Mineral-rich organic soil supports healthy, prolific plants. Such healthy plants do not require artificial pesticides. Thus, we can reduce the threat by pesticides to public health.

Cities must treat and recycle sewage to farms. This can be done on a local level by using composting toilets, which decompose food scraps as well as excrement. Urban individuals should take the initiative by installing composting toilets, and ceasing to use the sewage systems.

Obviously, eating for the environment means eating and recycling organically-grown produce as much as possible. The use of pesticides encourages mono-cropping with single food crops year after year. This leads to soil erosion and land being turned to desert. About one-third of the Earth's landmass is suffering desertification as a result of overgrazing, overcultivation, improper irrigation, deforestation and lack of reforestation. By eating a minimum or no meat you are taking your money out of the hands of the main contributor to gobal destruction: livestock production. By eating organically or biodynamically grown produce, you are placing your money in the hands of farmers who care for the health of the soil. By eating fruit, you are encouraging the planting of trees. We desperately need more trees to help stabilise the Earth's climate and avert global warming.

Global warming is creating serious, potentially catastrophic, climatic changes. CO_2 and methane emissions are major contributors to global warming. About two-thirds of CO_2 emissions are created by burning fossil fuels. The EarthSave Foundation estimates that 78 kilojoules of fossil fuel are expended to produce one kilojoule of protein from beef. Only 2 kilojoules are needed to produce 1 kilojoule of protein from soybeans. The amount of CO_2 produced in providing the average American family with beef for one year is about the same as the CO_2 produced by their car in six months! 20 per cent of the world's methane comes out of the rear end of cattle (EarthSave Foundation 1992). In Central America cattle-ranching has destroyed more rainforest than any other activity. Additionally, 90 per cent of the new cattle ranches in the Amazon go out of business in less than eight years, their soil base depleted from overgrazing. To create grazing land for cattle 25 per cent of Central American rainforests have been cleared (EarthSave Foundation 1992).

Fruit skin is the ultimate in biodegradable packaging. By eating fruit you can minimise your garbage, and save some trees from being killed for paper production. Take plastic carry-bags back to your greengrocer, and reuse them—better still, buy cloth or string bags.

By eating unmutilated living foods you can eliminate all your energy consumption associated with the use of kitchens. Minimal refrigeration may be necessary to preserve green-leaf vegetables and some fruits. However, the Symbiotic must eat living food at ambient temperature, and avoid the energy drain on the body-mind created by eating chilled food. So, if you use a refrigerator, remove your food from it several hours before the food is eaten. Warm your fruit in the sun if possible.

Houses without kitchens have a much lower energy requirement, and can easily be run on solar power in most parts of the world.

The way of the Symbiotic is profoundly ecological. It demands and provides your deep integration into the Earth's network of ecological interconnections. Nature flows through your body-mind in the form of food.

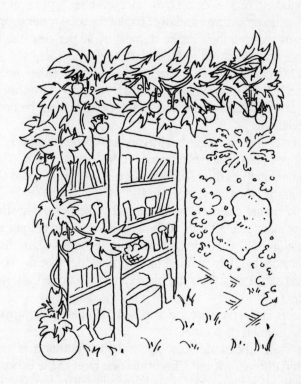

Eating for a
New Society

V ast amounts of land, water and energy are required to produce meat. In the United States over one-third of all raw materials consumed for all purposes are devoted to the production of livestock. Livestock consume 70 per cent of the total US grain production and over half of the total water supply. If Americans reduced their intake of meat by 10 per cent, the freed resources could be used to feed 100 000 000 people.

Government agricultural programmes and subsidies must be redirected from supporting animal and feed farms to fruit and vegetable growers. Agricultural and health policies must be brought into alignment.

As a result of meat eating, health care has become a disaster, with over 10 per cent of some countries' GNP devoted to it. The US government ignores their Surgeon-General's statement that 68 per cent of all diseases are diet related.

The following diseases and ailments can be positively affected by a low-meat diet: arthritis, asthma, breast cancer, colon cancer, constipation, diabetes, diverticulosis, gallstones, heart disease, hypertension, hypoglycaemia, impotence, kidney disease, obesity, osteoporosis, peptic ulcers, prostate cancer, salmonellosis, stroke, trichinosis.

There is now pressure on medical schools to improve the nutrition training of doctors.

Meanwhile, the understanding of better nutrition is rapidly spreading through society. This is just one facet of the ecocultural revolution among humanity. Soon humanity will understand 'green shit and amber skin' is a formula for health (assuming normal liver function and Caucasian ancestry). It is simply a sign of consumption of enough chlorophyll and beta-carotene foods.

An enormous social effort goes into the growth, distribution and preparation of toxic foods. Consequently, an equally enormous social effort goes into the production and supply of medicine and so-called health services. When you are not sick, you may still be sold medicines in your food. Animal foods contain sulfa drugs, tetracyclines and other antibiotics (EarthSave Foundation 1992).

Western medicine focuses on how to treat the symptoms of illnesses created by a mainly meat and grain diet. Chinese medicine focuses on how to treat the symptoms of illnesses created by a mainly rice diet. With Symbiotics, the food is the medicine. Thesis, antithesis, synthesis: a new symbiotic society bursts from the dialectic bubble.

The health and other social and environmental costs of disease-provoking foods should be borne by individuals in proportion to their consumption of them. When we have a 'fat and cholesterol tax', a 'protein and phosphorus tax' and a 'sucrose and caffeine tax' to cover the true costs of food abuse, there will be a new dawn of hope for us all.

Fruit-growing is three-dimensional permaculture (sustainable agriculture), rising above the two-dimensional agriculture of the past. The vertical dimension of trees provides more productive space than the merely horizontal fields. When society makes the shift to a symbiotic lifestyle, fruit will be abundant. One hectare of prime land can provide 250 kg of beef or 20 000 kg apples (Earth-Save Foundation 1992). We may even get more of our greens from vines and trees: grape, lime and bay leaves are edible. There will be enough food for everyone. The world will be released from the time, effort, stress, and premature mortality of the food–medicine dialectic. There will be effortless creation of paradise on Earth and tribalisation of space—Mother Earth awaits our caring, Father Sky awaits our daring.

Peace, social development, creativity, knowledge, understanding, personal growth and happiness are natural pursuits of healthy body-minds. Each person is free to choose to join the planetary symbiotic celebration that has already begun to enliven the Earth! If you are responsible, you will have the ability to respond positively to this choice.

Eating for the Future

If developing countries continue to take on high-meat diets and developed countries do not drastically reduce meat consumption, there will be a full ecological catastrophe. Topsoil depletion has caused many great civilisations to collapse—but it has never yet occurred on a global scale. Food consumers must rapidly reduce their meat consumption and farmers must switch to substainable agriculture. Besides organic food, farmers can grow flax and hemp for paper and cloth production, and tree crops for biomass fuel.

Like nuclear energy, genetic engineering harbours both power and danger. We must forestall its use until we have a very deep understanding of the dangers. We must not allow commercial interests to override ecological needs.

Commercial interests are trying to introduce transgenic foods: foods containing genes from different species, such as a tomato containing some genes from a pig (Gasser & Fraley 1992). These transgenic species are new organisms. They lack subtle symbiotic attunement, and will ultimately disrupt ecosystems. Everything in the ecosphere is interconnected in a web of symbiotic relations, and the introduction of transgenic species is bound to be disruptive, unpredictable and fraught with danger.

Nevertheless, adopting a symbiotic lifestyle must not mean becoming a complete victim of the Earth's ecosystem. Bacteria or viruses may yet evolve to create new diseases that our immune systems cannot handle (such as HIV). Surrender to the forces of nature must be balanced by empowerment through influencing nature. We will have to take increasing control of our ecosystem in the future. This is already beginning with simple ecosystems for spacecraft, and this will continue to be a driving force for our understanding.

Even now we are developing the ability to control our genetic basis. Evolution will eventually become 'prevolution'—selection of the most creative symbiotic system. In the distant future, as we creatively redesign ourselves we must also redesign our food, but always maintaining the essential symbiotic relationship.

Earthly evolution is leading us into interstellar prevolution of ourselves in complete symbiotic systems. Who knows, maybe we will end up as the symbiotic riders of dolphins swimming in the weightless atmosphere of interstellar space craft? The deep future will take no heed of our present religious, cultural, historical, technological or planetary context. Ultimately, our present symbiotic context will be lost in the infinite.

Eating for Love

The cascade of your colours calls out to me from the garden. I am drawn to you incessantly, like waves always fresh in their seeking of the sand. With my hands I feel your soft rounded skin, and intuitively I know that you are ripe. My fingers work gently to peel away your outer layer. Juice begins to trickle between my fingers, and my lips rush to savour your sweetness. Waterfalls of sensation run down my throat and send fulfilment to my outer reaches. We are inseparable, bound together by the genetic artistry of aeons. We are perfect for each other. One's most natural giving is a response to the other's deepest need.

This symbiotic harmony, this laughter of the heart, can be none other than love itself.

2

What
to
Eat?

Recipes

These recipes are your launching pad for your travels as a Symbiotic into the CaPNaK galaxy. I have indicated the acid–alkaline and yin–yang effect of each recipe; you can also check these on the CaPNaK Chart. If either acid–alkaline or yin–yang is not mentioned, then the combination is balanced in that dimension. The possibilities of live-food combinations and presentation are only limited by your willingness to experiment.

Prepared live foods must be eaten as soon as possible, especially when the food has been blended or juiced.

Fruit Salads

Acidic Exciter Fruit Salad
(1 serving)
Moderately acid–yin

1 banana, sliced

1 cup peaches, sliced

½ cup nectarines, sliced

1 tsp pumpkin seeds, ground

1 tsp unhulled sesame seeds, ground

1 tsp sunflower seeds, ground

Mix, and serve.

Alkaline Feast Fruit Salad
(1 serving)
Moderately alkaline–yin

2 oranges

400 g papaya

4 fresh figs

Dice, mix, and serve.

Apple Adventure
(1 serving)
Moderately yin

2 ripe apples

1 kiwi fruit

ground cinnamon, cloves and
  nutmeg to taste

*Warm the fruit in sunlight (but
no more than two hours). Chop
the apples into fingers, and finely
chop the apple seeds. Remove the
hard end of the kiwi fruit, rub off
the hairs, and with the skin intact
cut the fruit into thin slices. Mix
the fruit, seeds, and spices, and
serve immediately.*

Chinese Pears
(1 serving)
Moderately yin

2 ripe pears

1 fig (if dried, then presoak)

$1/8$ tsp ground cinnamon

$1/8$ tsp ground nutmeg

*Finely chop the fig, and mix
with the spices. Remove the top
two-thirds of the cores of the
pears. Fill the cavities with the fig
and spice mixture, and serve
immediately.*

Cold Evening Fruit Salad
(1 serving)
Moderately acid, strongly yin

$1/2$ avocado

4 bananas

ground cinnamon (optional)

*Mash together, and add cinnamon
if desired.*

Cold Morning Fruit Salad
(1 serving)
Slightly acid, strongly yin

4 bananas, sliced

400 g grapes, seeded

Mix.

Digger's Lunch Fruit Salad
(1 serving)
Slightly alkaline, moderately yin

1 large mango

2 oranges

4 apricots

1 bunch grapes

Chop and mix, or eat whole.

Melon Mix Fruit Salad
(3 servings)
Slightly acid–yin

$1/2$ watermelon

1 cantaloupe (rockmelon)

1 honeydew melon

Chop, and mix.

Strawberries Cardinal
(2 servings)
Moderately yin–acid

$1^1/_3$ cups strawberries, sliced

$1/_3$ cup orange juice, freshly
squeezed

$1/_2$ cup raspberries

Marinate the strawberries in orange juice for 1–4 hours. Puree the raspberries in a blender or food processor, and press through a sieve or colander to remove the seeds.

To serve, drain the strawberries, place in compotes or wineglasses, and top with raspberry sauce. Drink the juice.

Summer Breakfast Fruit Salad
(1 serving)
Slightly acid–yin

1 banana

4 peaches

1 pear

1 bunch grapes, seeded

lemon juice

Chop into pieces, mix and sprinkle with juice.

Yellow Snack Fruit Salad
(2 servings)
Slightly alkaline, moderately yin

1 papaya

$1/_2$ pineapple

lime or lemon juice

Chop, and sprinkle with juice.

Juices

Use a juice extractor or blender. Stir as much pulp as possible back into your juice: chew your juice! If the pulp is not returned, the juice will be more acidic than indicated below. Use unpeeled fruit whenever it is appropriate.

Green Juices (1–2 servings):

Thirst-quencher Juice
Strongly alkaline–yang

2 celery tops

greens from 1 beet

greens from 1 turnip

1 bunch watercress

Inner Peace Juice
Alkaline

200 g any greens

2 medium carrots

1 tomato

handful of parsley

Agro Juice
Strongly yang

50 g spinach
50 g beetroot
100 g carrot

Other Juices (1–2 servings):

Sweet Life Juice
Moderately acid–yin

1 cup alfalfa sprouts
$1^{1}/_{2}$ cups pineapple juice

Jumping Jack Juice
Moderately acid–yang

100 g carrot
50 g cucumber
50 g beetroot

Smoothies

Fruit Cup Smoothie
Moderately yin; banana strongly yin

200 g fruit juice (e.g. orange, apple or grape)
1 cup of any of the following: strawberries, pineapple, peaches, pears, papaya, banana

Tropical Smoothie
Moderately yin

1 banana
200 g coconut milk
1 tbsp carob powder

Business Juice
Slightly yang

1 beetroot
3 chicory leaves
1 spring onion
1 radish (discard the top)
150 g carrot

Brain Juice
Slightly yin

1 large bunch of grapes
1 pear

Instant Happiness Juice
Moderately alkaline–yin

100 g orange segments
50 g apricot
50 g grapes

Desert Night Smoothie
Moderately acid, strongly yin

200 g apple juice
1 banana
¼ cup dates, pitted

Thinker's Smoothie
Moderately acid, strongly yin

2 cups pineapple juice
1 banana
2 cups strawberries

Vegetable Dips and Soups

Soups may be made from blends of vegetables and/or juices. If you wish, warm them to no more than 50°C (122°F) (higher heat will kill the enzymes). Eat as soon as possible for maximum nutrition.

Guacamole Dip
(serves 4 dippers)
Strongly acid–yin

2 or 3 avocados, mashed

1 tomato, mashed (include skin)

1 tbsp kelp or 1 stalk celery, finely chopped

$^1/_2$ onion, chopped

$^1/_4$ cup chillies

juice of 2 lemons

1 clove garlic, crushed

Mix well, or blend and serve.

Asparagus Soup
(2 servings)
Moderately acid–yin

400 g asparagus

1 stalk celery, chopped, or 1 tbsp kelp

1 tbsp parsley, chopped

pinch of oregano and thyme

2 tbsp ground almonds

water (warm in winter) according to taste

Blend, and serve.

Cabbage Soup
(2 servings)
Moderately acid

1 cup carrot juice

1 cup celery juice

1 cup cabbage, shredded

1 red pepper (capsicum), chopped

1 tomato, chopped (include skin)

$^1/_2$ avocado, chopped

$^1/_2$ tsp cayenne pepper

Blend, adding avocado last.

Cream of Spinach Soup
(2 servings)
Moderately alkaline–yang

400 g spinach, chopped

$^1/_4$ avocado

$^1/_4$ cup onion

$^1/_4$ cup celery

pinch of your favourite herbs

2 cups water (warm in winter)

Blend, and serve.

Vegetable Soup
(3 servings)
Moderately acid

2 cups carrots, chopped

2 cups peas

2 stalks celery, chopped

1–3 cloves garlic, peeled and chopped

$1/2$ avocado

water (warm in winter) according to taste

Blend, and serve. Top with alfalfa sprouts.

Fruit Soups

Blend any good combination of fruits together to make fruit soup. For good digestion, a fruit soup is best eaten on its own.

Apricot and Banana Soup
(1 serving)
Slightly acid, strongly yin

4 apricots

1 banana

Blend, and serve.

Banana and Orange Soup
(1 serving)
Slightly acid, moderately yin

1 banana

1 orange

$1/2$ cup orange juice

Blend, and serve.

Orange and Apple Soup
(1 serving)
Slightly yin

1 orange, peeled

1 apple

lemon juice, to taste

$1/2$ cup orange juice

Blend, and serve.

Spicy Soup
(3 servings)
Strongly acid–yin

2 cups apples, chopped

2 cups bananas, sliced

1 cup raisins, soaked

$1/2$ cup unhulled sesame seeds (tahini), ground

$1/2$ cup ground sunflower seeds

pinch of nutmeg or cinnamon

squeeze of lemon juice

2 cups of apple juice

Blend, and serve.

Vegetable Salads

Nut butters or whole nuts and seeds can be used as dressings or garnishes. Squeeze juice from citrus fruits onto salads to reduce their rate of oxidation (browning) after being chopped. Again, eat salads freshly prepared for maximum nutrition.

Lunch Salad
(1 serving)
Moderately alkaline

1 cup green lettuce leaves

$1/_2$ cup red cabbage, shredded

$1/_4$ cup turnip, shredded

$1/_4$ cup summer squash (zucchini), chopped

$1/_4$ cup lentils, sprouted

Make a bed of lettuce leaves, add the other ingredients (mixed) on top.

Quick Coleslaw
(1 serving)
Moderately alkaline–yang

$1/_2$ cup carrot, grated

$1/_2$ cup white cabbage, grated

$1/_2$ cup celery, chopped

$1/_4$ cup parsley, chopped

$1/_2$ cup apple, diced

Mix, and serve.

Summer Salad
(1 serving)
Moderately alkaline, strongly yang

200 g spinach leaves

2 stalks celery, diced

1 bunch watercress

1 cup grated summer squash (zucchini)

$1/_2$ cup red onion rings

$1/_2$ cup mushrooms, sliced

Mix, and serve.

Vegetable Nut Loaf
(2 servings)
Slightly alkaline, moderately yang

1 cup carrots, grated

1 cup tomatoes, chopped

1 cup celery, grated

$1/_2$ cup parsley, chopped

$1/_2$ cup green capsicum, grated

2 tbsp hulled sesame seeds (tahini)

1 clove garlic, crushed

Add enough ground nuts to hold it together. Mould into shape, and garnish with herbs or seeds.

Winter Salad
(1 serving)
Moderately yin

1 cup broccoli, chopped

$^1/_2$ cup winter squash, sliced

$^1/_2$ cup butternut pumpkin, grated

1 avocado, diced

3 lettuce leaves

*Make a bed of lettuce leaves; add
the other ingredients (mixed).*

Sandwich, Platter, Tacos

Paradise Leaf Sandwich
(4 servings)
Moderately acid–yin

3 avocados

1 pineapple

10 broccoli and/or lettuce leaves

*Chop fruit into bite-size chunks,
mix, and roll up in leaves.*

Pineapple Platter
(3 servings)
Moderately acid–strongly yin

1 pineapple

2 avocados

30 dates, pitted and crushed

*Cut pineapple in 15 mm thick
slices; spread slices with avocado,
and top with crushed dates.*

Tacos
(1 serving)
Moderately acid–yin

1 avocado, mashed

1 cup mixed sprouts

3 tbsp orange juice

1 tbsp unhulled sesame seeds
(tahini)

4 tender cabbage leaves (for taco
'shells')

Mix, and serve in cabbage leaves.

Cheese, Bread and Cereal

Fermented Seed Cheese
(2 servings)
Sunflower is strongly acid–yin; unhulled sesame is strongly alkaline

$1/2$ cup sunflower and/or sesame seeds

1 cup water

Blend seeds and water into a creamy sauce. Cover the mixture loosely in a porcelain or glass container, and put it in a warm place or in the sun. Leave to ferment for 5–9 hours. Cover, and refrigerate to stop fermentation.

Best served with salads. Eat in moderation. Fermented foods are a source of vitamin B_{12}.

Sprouted Cereal
(4 servings)
Strongly acid, moderately yin

2 cups sprouted grain (from 1 cup of seeds: wheat, rye, barley, etc.)

cold water

Sprout the grain by soaking in cold water for 8 hours. Then rinse every six hours until the roots shoot. Taste the sprouted grain, and continue rinsing every 6 hours until it is soft enough to chew.

Eat this cereal with salads, dried fruits and nuts as a muesli, or on its own.

Adding dried fruit is not a recommended food combination.

Sun Bread
(4 servings)
Strongly acid, moderately yin

2 cups sprouted grain (from 1 cup of seeds; wheat, rye, barley, etc.)

cold water

Sprout the grain by soaking in cold water for 8 hours, then rinsing every six hours until the roots shoot. Mill or press the grain to make a dough. Press the dough and cut into wafers 5–10 mm thick. Place in a warm spot or in the sun to dry. Turn the bread wafers with a spatula to dry the other side.

You must chew this cereal food very thoroughly for good digestion. The Sun Bread is strongly acidic, and should be eaten in moderation; eat it with a strongly alkaline salad.

Do not eat Sun Bread for at least 30 minutes after eating fruit, to allow fruit to leave the enzyme-stomach to avoid fermentation (see Eating for Digestion). Do not eat fruit for at least 2 hours after eating Sun Bread.

Variations: Seeds and/or seasonings may be added before pressing the dough. Dried fruit may be added, but this is not a recommended food combination. See Eating for Digestion for information on food combining.

The CaPNaK Chart
in Detail

This chapter will provide you with more in-depth information about the structure and use of the CaPNaK Chart. It is not essential to read this, but it will provide you with more skill and understanding. You may wish to review What Does It All Mean before proceeding.

The horizontal direction of the CaPNaK Chart (left/right) shows the residual potassium or sodium provided by each food after subtracting the body's balanced ratio (potassium to sodium, 12:1) of these minerals.

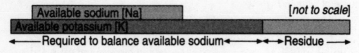

Potassium-residue in an orange.

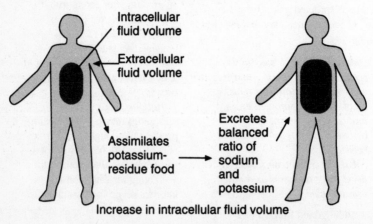

Change in fluid balance an hour or two after eating potassium-residue food.

Similarly, the vertical direction of the CaPNaK Chart (up/down) shows the residual calcium or phosphorus provided by each food after subtracting the body's balanced ratio (calcium to phosphorus, 1:1).

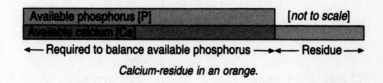

← Required to balance available phosphorus —→ ←— Residue —→

Calcium-residue in an orange.

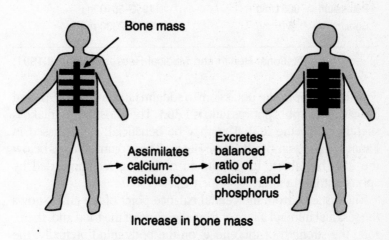

Change in bone mass after eating calcium-residue foods.

To construct the CaPNaK Chart I have used a potassium to sodium balance ratio of 12:1, and a calcium to phosphorus balance ratio of 1:1. My own experience of the balance in temperate, subtropical and tropical climates and seasons indicates that the balance ratios I have used here are a good compromise. You can shift the balance point you use on the CaPNaK Chart as discussed in Eating for the Climate and Eating for the Seasons.

A sample day's eating for a Symbiotic might include:

4 sticks of celery (70 g each stick)	6 large oranges (190 g each)
500 g broccoli (1½ heads)	20 g unhulled tahini (sesame
5 bananas (100 g each)	seeds)

This recommended daily (dietary) intake (RDI) would provide:

		RDI
Calcium	1218 mg	800–1000 mg
Phosphorus	897 mg	1000 mg
Potassium	6661 mg	1950–5640 mg
Sodium	515 mg	920–2300 mg

(National Health and Medical Research Council 1991)

In this example, the potassium to sodium ratio is then 12.9:1, and the calcium to phosphorus ratio is 1.36:1. The phosphorus intake is slightly below the RDI. This may be beneficial, as discussed in Eating for Bones and Soft Tissue Health. The sodium intake is below the RDI, but above the minimum of 500 mg recommended by sports-nutrition expert Dr Robert Haas (1983).

The distance from the central balance point of the chart shows the residual mineral left over from digestion of the food and, therefore, the strength of the effects on the body-mind. Actually, the above is strictly true only in the central linear region. You can distinguish this region on the complete chart by its shading.

There is a logarithmic region around the periphery of the CaPNaK Chart. The distances inside the central rectangle are linear, and the co-ordinates are logarithmic outside this rectangular region.

On the potassium–sodium (horizontal) axis the scale of the rectangular linear region goes between plus and minus 3 mg per gram. Outside the linear region on this horizontal axis the logarithmic scale goes to 10, 100, etc., at succeeding gradations.

On the calcium–phosphorus (vertical) axis the scale of the rectangular linear region goes between plus and minus 0.3 mg per

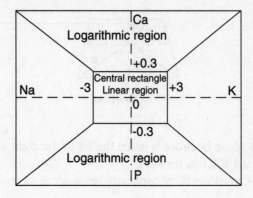

Linear and logarithmic regions of the CaPNaK Chart.

gram. Outside the linear region on this vertical axis the logarithmic scale goes to 1, then 10 at succeeding gradations.

This means, for example, that celery (see the CaPNaK Chart on page 166) is ten times stronger in sodium-residue than its position would imply if the scale was entirely linear. This is why only 280 g celery is enough to balance the potassium-residue in the example given on p. 162. You must assign more strength to the effects of foods outside the rectangular region.

You can balance the CaPNaK minerals with three or more foods, as shown below.

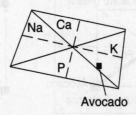

Avocado

The chart is tilted to one corner as avocado is eaten.

Result: Overdose of potassium (K) and phosphorus (P); acid–yin state of body-mind.

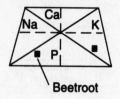

Beetroot

Then as some beetroot is eaten the tilt to the right is corrected, but the chart still tilts forward.

Result: Overdose of phosphorus remains; acid state of body-mind.

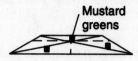

Finally, by eating mustard greens, the tilt forward is rebalanced, and the chart returns to the horizontal.

Result: No overdose remains; balanced state of body-mind.

Alternatively, you can visualise the balancing process as arrows (vectors):

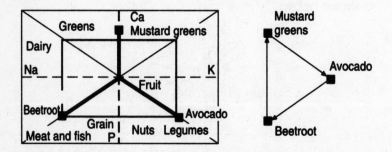

Note that the arrows for beetroot and mustard greens are lengthened compared with their length on the chart. This is because a larger quantity of beetroot is eaten. Mustard greens are well into the logarithmic region of the chart, so this is shown with a lengthened arrow.

You can use this vector method on the chart, using a thumb and forefinger. Just span the distances with your hand so that you walk your hand around the chart. The directions and distances are given by the locations of the foods you eat relative to the origin (central balance point). Span out the distance of a food from the balance point, and add that to your current position on the chart. Adjust the span, taking into account the relative quantities of the foods and whether they are in the logarithmic region. For example, if there is twice the weight of one food compared with another, then its arrow should be doubled in length. Your current position on the chart represents your body-mind state resulting from the foods eaten and your starting body-mind state.

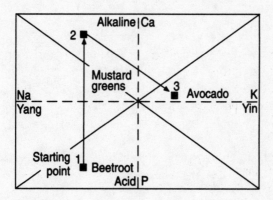

Detailed Explanation of CaPNaK Balance

The body-mind regulates sodium and potassium in precise concentrations in the fluids inside and outside the cells: the intracellular and extracellular fluids (Bronner & Comar 1960). There is a higher concentration of sodium in the extracellular fluid and a higher concentration of potassium in the intracellular fluid.

If your body-mind absorbs extra sodium and potassium, then your body-mind regulates the concentrations by moving water,

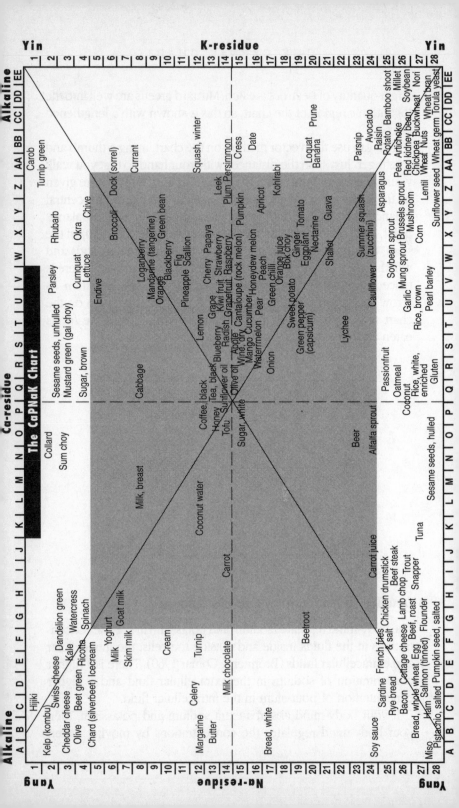

Art Cards   **by Carol Pessin**

My cards are unique because each one is an
original hand painted art work using water
colors and Sumi ink with envelopes matching
the design of the theme.

I study the Japanese brush painting technique
(Sumi-e) and add my own creative energy and
love which I derive from all people.

My art continues with calligraphy, Ikebana
(flower arranging), Sumi ink painting on rice
paper and art work on floors, walls, carpets,
glass, slate and I tell my husband to keep
moving or I'll paint on him.

White Plains, N.Y.
(914)328-0544 fax(914)328-4492
e-mail:KAROLV23@aol.com
web:www.carolartcards.com

Food Index

Alfalfa sprout O24
Almond see Nuts
Apple S15
Apricot Y16
Artichoke BB26
Asparagus Y25
Avocado BB24

Bacon C26
Bamboo shoot CC25
Banana AA20
Barley see Pearl barley
Bean see Pearl barley;
  Red kidney bean
Beef: roast G25;
  steak I25
Beer O23
Beet green C4
Beetroot F20
Blackberry V10
Blueberry S14
Bok choy W18
Brazil nut see Nuts
Bread: white A17;
  whole wheat B27;
  see also Rye bread
Broccoli X6
Brussels sprout Y26
Buckwheat CC27
Butter B13

Cabbage Q8
Cantaloupe (rockmelon) T15
Capsicum see Green pepper
Carob AA1
Carrot I14
Carrot juice I24
Cashew see Nuts

Cauliflower U24
Celery C12
Chard (silverbeet) B5
Cheddar see Cheddar
Cheese see Cheddar
  cheese; Cottage cheese;
  Ricotta cheese; Swiss
  cheese
Cherry V13
Chestnut see Nuts
Chicken drumstick H25
Chickpea AA27
Chilli see Green chilli
Chive Y4
Chocolate see Milk
  chocolate
Coconut Q26
Coconut water K12
Coffee, black P13
Collard N2
Corn X27
Cottage cheese E26
Cream F10
Cress BB15
Cucumber T16
Cumquat V4
Currant AA8

Dandelion green F3
Date BB16
Dock (sorrel) Z6

Egg E27
Eggplant W19
Endive U5

Fig W11
Flounder G27

French fries & salt E25

Gai choy see Mustard green
Garlic U26
Ginger W19
Gluten R28
Goat milk G7
Grape U13
Grapefruit U14
Greenbean X10
Green chilli U17
Green pepper
  (capsicum) S19
Guava Y4

Ham C27
Hazelnut see Nuts
Hijiki C1
Honey P13
Honeydew melon V16

Icecream E5

Kale E3
Kelp (kombu) A2
Kiwi fruit U14
Kohlrabi Z18

Lamb chop G26
Leek Z14
Lemon T12
Lentil Z27
Lettuce V4
Loganberry V8
Loquat AA20
Lychee T22

Mandarine (tangerine) V9

Mango S16
Margarine B12
Melon see Cantaloupe;
  Honeydew melon
Milk: breast L8; full-cream E6;
  goat see Goat milk;
  skim E7
Milk chocolate D14
Millet EE26
Miso A28
Mung sprout V26
Mushroom Y26
Mustard green (gai choy) Q3

Nectarine X20
Nori sheet EE27
Nuts (almond, Brazil nut,
  cashew, chestnut,
  hazelnut, peanut, pecan,
  pine nut, walnut) BB27;
  see also Pistachio

Oatmeal Q26
Okra X4
Olive B4
Olive oil Q15
Onion R17
Orange U9
Orange juice V18

Papaya W13
Parsley V2
Parsnip BB23
Passionfruit Q25
Pea AA26
Peach V17
Peanut see Nuts
Pear U16

Pearl barley U28
Pecan see Nuts
Persimmon AA14
Pine nut see Nuts
Pineapple U11
Pistachio, salted B28
Plum Z14
Potato BB25
Prune CC20
Pumpkin Y15
Pumpkin seed, salted E28

Radish S14
Raisin BB25
Raspberry W14
Red kidney bean AA26
Rhubarb X2
Rice: brown T27;
  white, enriched Q27
Ricotta cheese E4
Rockmelon see Cantaloupe
Rye bread C25

Salmon (tinned) D27
Sardines C25
Scallion W11
Sesame seeds: hulled M28;
  unhulled Q2
Shallot W21
Skim milk see Milk
Snapper I27
Sorrel see Dock
Soy sauce A24
Soybean EE2
Soybean sprout V25
Spinach G4
Sprouts see Alfalfa sprout;

Mung sprout; Soybean
  sprout
Squash: summer W24;
  winter AA12
Strawberry W14
Sugar: brown Q4; white P15
Sum choy N3
Summer squash (zucchini)
  see Squash
Sunflower oil P14
Sunflower seed Y28
Sweet potato T19
Swiss cheese D2

Tangerine see Mandarine
Tea, black P13
Tofu O14
Tomato Y19
Torula yeast DD28
Trout I26
Tuna K27
Turnip F12
Turnip green AA2

Walnut see Nuts
Watercress G4
Watermelon S16
Wheat AA2
Wheat bran DD28
Wheat germ BB28
Wine, dry S15
Winter squash see Squash

Yeast see Torula yeast
Yoghurt F6

Zucchini see Squash,
  summer

sodium and potassium in or out of the cells. Also, concentrations are regulated by excreting water, sodium and potassium. The actual physiological mechanisms by which your body-mind achieves this regulation are complex and numerous. However, the resulting principle is that for any ratio of the volumes of intracellular to extracellular fluids there is a corresponding ratio of dissolved potassium to sodium in the body-mind. This is an approximation of the function of the complex systems and structures of the body-mind, of value for its practical use, rather than its physiological accuracy.

Many conditions and symptoms of the body-mind relate to the ratio of the volumes of intracellular to extracellular fluids in the body. These symptoms are adjusted, through the ratio of the fluids, by changing the ratio of potassium to sodium in your body.

The changes in this ratio of potassium to sodium in your body can be related to the residual potassium or sodium provided by a food. The residue is the sodium or potassium left after this ratio is subtracted from the absorbed (eaten) potassium and sodium. For those so inclined, a mathematical explanation is given on page 169. The CaPNaK Chart was constructed using these equations.

Potassium and sodium are two of the four main food minerals. The other two are the ubiquitous minerals, calcium and phosphorus. There is a higher proportion of calcium in your bones, and a higher proportion of phosphorus in your tissues.

Phosphates dissolved in your body fluids are acidic, whereas calcium's effect is alkaline. Another source of acidity is uric acid from the metabolising of protein. If you do not eat excessive quantities of protein, other sources of acidity and alkalinity are minor, and the absorbed (eaten) calcium and phosphorus affect the acid–alkaline balance.

Your body-mind precisely regulates the acid–alkaline balance in the blood within a narrow range of pH. If extra calcium and phosphorus are absorbed into your blood, then your body-mind regulates the pH by moving calcium and phosphorus in or out of your bones and tissues. The pH is also regulated by the excretion of calcium and phosphorus from your body–mind. The basic principle is that the disturbance of the ratio of calcium to phosphorus in the blood is regulated by varying the mineral densities of calcium and phosphorus in the bones and tissues.

Again, this principle is an approximation of the function of the complex systems and structures of the body-mind, of its value for its practical use, rather than its physiological accuracy.

Many conditions and symptoms of your body-mind relate to the mineral densities of calcium and phosphorus in your bones and tissues. These symptoms and conditions are adjusted, through the mineral densities, by regulating the ratio of calcium to phosphorus in your blood.

Disturbances in this ratio of calcium to phosphorus in your blood are related to the residual calcium or phosphorus provided by a food. The residue is the calcium or phosphorus left after this ratio is subtracted from the absorbed (eaten) calcium and phosphorus.

The CaPNaK Equations

The transformation equations for determining the co-ordinates of a food on the CaPNaK Chart are:

$$K_{res} = \Delta K - \left(\frac{K}{Na}\right)\Delta Na \qquad \text{(Equation 1)}$$

where K_{res} is the residual potassium; $K/Na = 12$ is the mean equilibrium ratio of potassium to sodium required by the body; ΔK is the potassium, and ΔNa is the sodium provided by the food.

$$Ca_{res} = \Delta Ca - \left(\frac{Ca}{P}\right)\Delta P \qquad \text{(Equation 2)}$$

where Ca_{res} is the residual calcium; $Ca/P = 1.0$ is the mean equilibrium ratio of calcium to phosphorus required by the body; ΔCa is the calcium, and ΔP is the phosphorus provided by the food. A sodium- or phosphorus-residue is expressed as a negative potassium- or calcium-residue, respectively.

Food Composition Data

Perfect meal balancing should not be your aim. You must develop awareness of the current state of your body-mind and the state you wish to be in after the meal. Then you can determine the shift in body-mind state you want the meal to provide, and choose the foods accordingly.

To do your own calculations of the residues for the foods in the food composition table, follow this simple example of a meal consisting of 100 g avocado, 150 g beetroot and 50 g mustard greens.

1 Multiply each food's K-res and Ca-res amounts in the table by the weight of the food, and add up each column, e.g.

	K-res	mg	Ca-res	mg
Avocado	5.56 x 100 =	556.0	−0.32 x 100 =	−32.0
Beetroot	−3.85 x 150 =	−577.5	−0.17 x 150 =	−25.5
Mustard greens	−0.07 x 50 =	−3.5	1.33 x 50 =	66.5
Total		**−25.0**		**9.0**

The K-res and Ca-res values for each food in the table are the co-ordinates on the CaPNaK Chart. The negative sign indicates a deficit, and the positive sign a surplus.

2 To turn a negative K-res value into the corresponding positive Na-res value, divide by 12. For the sample meal above, −25.0 mg K-res ÷ 12 = 2.25 mg Na-res.

3 A negative Ca-res converts directly to a positive P-res; the Ca-res for avocado is −32.0 mg, so the P-res is 32.0 mg.

According to the residue totals, this meal will produce a slightly yang–alkaline shift in your body-mind.

The columns on the right in the following table give the amounts of the four minerals in 100 g of each food. The food composition data is derived mainly from the *Nutrition Almanac* (Nutrition Search 1979). For the mathematically minded, see my equations for the conversion of mineral amounts to residue values in mg/g (p. 169).

Food	Residues (mg/g)		Mineral amounts (mg/100 g)			
	K-res	Ca-res	Ca	P	Na	K
Dairy products						
Cheeses						
Cheddar cheese	−74.43	2.36	753.6	517.9	628.6	100.0
Cottage cheese	−47.78	−0.82	68.6	150.4	406.2	96.0
Ricotta cheese	−9.05	0.49	206.9	158.1	84.1	104.5
Swiss cheese	−30.61	3.61	971.4	610.7	264.3	110.7
Milks						
Milk, breast	−1.43	0.19	32.5	13.0	16.2	51.9
Milk, full cream	−4.46	0.26	119.3	93.4	49.2	143.9
Milk, goat	−3.95	0.23	133.6	110.7	50.0	204.5
Milk, skim	−4.51	0.22	123.3	100.8	51.4	165.7
Other dairy products						
Chocolate, milk	−7.68	0.00	232.1	232.1	96.4	389.3
Cream	−3.60	0.13	93.3	80.0	40.0	120.0
Icecream	−8.53	0.32	132.3	100.8	87.2	193.2
Yoghurt	−4.00	0.26	120.7	94.7	46.3	154.6
Drinks						
Beer	−0.60	−0.25	5.0	30.0	7.1	25.0
Coffee, black	0.23	0.00	1.9	2.1	1.0	34.6
Tea, black	0.16	0.00	2.1	1.7	0.7	24.2
Wine, dry	0.32	−0.01	9.2	10.0	5.0	92.1
Fats, oils and condiments						
Butter	−118.19	0.04	19.8	15.9	986.8	22.9
Margarine	−118.10	0.07	21.1	14.1	985.9	21.1
Miso	−1590.57	−10.94	308.0	1402.0	13,381.0	1515.0

Food	Residues (mg/g)		Mineral amounts (mg/100 g)			
	K-res	Ca-res	Ca	P	Na	K
Olive oil	0.00	0.01	0.5	0.0	0.0	0.0
Soy sauce	−875.67	−0.22	83.3	105.6	7327.8	366.7
Sunflower oil	0.00	0.00	0.0	0.0	0.0	0.0
Tofu	−0.42	0.02	128.0	126.0	7.0	42.0
Yeast, torula	19.00	−13.07	428.6	1735.7	14.3	2071.4
Fruit						
Apple	0.88	−0.03	6.7	9.4	1.1	101.1
Apricot	2.54	−0.06	15.8	21.9	0.9	264.0
Avocado, pitted	5.56	−0.32	10.0	42.0	4.0	604.0
Banana	3.51	−0.18	8.0	26.0	1.3	366.7
Blackberry	1.62	0.13	31.9	18.8	0.7	170.1
Blueberry	0.72	0.02	15.2	13.1	0.7	80.7
Cantaloupe (rockmelon)	1.07	−0.02	14.0	16.0	12.0	251.0
Carob (Na and K values not found)	0.00	2.71	352.0	81.0	0.0	0.0
Cherry	1.53	0.03	20.0	16.9	1.5	171.5
Cumquat	1.60	0.40	60.0	20.0	5.0	220.0
Currant	3.36	0.20	60.0	40.0	3.0	372.0
Date, pitted	6.36	−0.04	59.0	63.0	1.0	648.0
Fig	1.70	0.13	35.0	22.0	2.0	194.0
Grape	1.19	0.04	15.7	11.8	3.3	158.2
Grapefruit	1.23	0.00	16.0	16.0	1.0	135.0
Guava	2.41	−0.19	23.0	42.0	4.0	289.0
Honeydew melon	1.07	−0.02	14.0	16.0	12.0	251.3
Kiwi fruit	1.39	0.03	18.0	15.3	1.3	155.3
Lemon	0.82	0.06	17.3	10.9	0.9	92.7
Loganberry	1.70	0.18	34.7	16.7	0.7	170.1
Loquat	1.70	−0.16	20.0	36.0	0.0	348.0
Lychee	0.78	−0.21	4.7	25.3	2.0	102.0
Mandarine (tangerine)	1.44	0.17	37.0	20.0	2.0	168.0
Mango	0.82	−0.02	7.7	10.0	5.3	145.7
Nectarine	2.07	−0.18	4.0	22.0	5.3	270.7
Olive, salted	−89.75	0.90	105.0	15.0	750.0	25.0
Orange	1.39	0.16	30.0	14.4	0.6	146.1

Food	Residues (mg/g)		Mineral amounts (mg/100 g)			
	K-res	Ca-res	Ca	P	Na	K
Orange juice	1.56	−0.10	12.0	22.0	2.0	180.0
Papaya	1.98	0.04	20.0	16.0	3.0	234.0
Passionfruit	0.12	−0.51	13.0	64.0	28.0	348.0
Peach	1.65	−0.09	7.8	16.5	0.9	175.7
Pear	1.06	−0.03	8.0	11.0	2.0	130.0
Persimmon	2.98	0.01	27.0	26.0	1.0	310.0
Pineapple	1.30	0.09	16.8	7.7	1.3	145.8
Plum	2.75	0.01	18.0	17.0	2.0	299.0
Prune	8.08	−0.17	90.0	107.0	11.0	940.0
Raisin	4.36	−0.39	61.8	101.2	27.3	763.0
Raspberry	1.59	0.00	22.0	22.0	0.8	168.3
Rhubarb	2.31	0.78	95.9	18.0	1.6	250.8
Strawberry	1.48	0.00	21.3	21.3	1.3	164.0
Watermelon	0.88	−0.03	7.0	10.0	1.0	100.0
Grains						
Barley, pearl	1.24	−1.73	16.0	189.0	3.0	160.0
Bread, rye	−65.35	−0.74	73.9	147.8	556.5	143.5
Bread, white	−60.00	−0.09	87.0	95.7	508.7	104.3
Bread, whole wheat	−60.39	−1.26	100.0	226.1	526.1	273.9
Buckwheat	6.44	−3.14	33.0	347.0	1.0	656.0
Corn	2.38	−2.06	16.9	222.9	0.8	248.3
Gluten	0.34	−1.00	40.0	140.0	2.1	60.0
Millet	11.76	−2.50	20.0	270.0	2.0	1200.0
Oatmeal	0.57	−0.48	9.2	57.1	0.3	60.8
Rice, brown	1.16	−1.88	32.7	220.4	8.2	214.3
Rice, white enriched	0.30	−0.70	24.1	93.8	5.1	91.8
Wheat	3.30	−3.31	40.8	371.7	3.3	370.0
Wheat bran	10.13	−11.56	118.9	1275.4	9.0	1121.1
Wheat germ	7.91	−10.46	72.0	1118.0	3.0	827.0
Legumes and sprouts						
Alfalfa sprout	−0.53	−0.30	18.0	48.0	9.0	55.0
Bean, green	1.55	0.13	56.4	43.6	7.3	242.7
Bean, red kidney	3.01	−1.02	37.8	140.0	3.2	340.0
Chickpea	4.85	−1.81	150.0	331.0	26.0	797.0

Food	Residues (mg/g)		Mineral amounts (mg/100 g)			
	K-res	Ca-res	Ca	P	Na	K
Lentil, raw	4.30	–2.98	79.0	377.0	30.0	790.0
Mung sprout	1.66	–0.45	19.0	63.8	4.8	222.9
Soybean, dry	16.17	–3.28	226.0	554.0	5.0	1677.0
Soybean sprout	1.92	–0.42	33.0	75.0	4.0	240.0
Meat and poultry						
Bacon	–80.22	–0.95	13.0	107.9	679.3	130.0
Beef, roast	–4.52	–1.50	10.8	161.0	60.8	277.8
Beef, steak	–3.37	–1.11	7.5	118.7	45.4	207.5
Chicken, drumstick	–6.37	–1.04	7.7	111.5	83.0	359.0
Egg	–11.82	–1.32	48.0	180.0	108.0	114.0
Ham	–87.91	–1.59	9.0	168.1	752.2	235.0
Lamb, chop	–3.65	–1.17	7.7	124.9	49.1	224.4
Nuts and seeds						
Almond	7.23	–2.70	233.8	504.2	4.2	773.2
Brazil nut	7.06	–5.07	185.7	692.9	0.7	715.0
Cashew	2.84	–3.35	37.9	372.9	15.0	464.3
Chestnut	3.79	–0.61	26.9	88.1	6.3	453.8
Coconut (meat)	–0.14	–0.83	12.5	95.0	22.5	256.3
Coconut milk (water)	–1.53	0.07	20.0	12.9	25.0	147.1
Hazelnut	6.77	–1.28	208.9	337.0	2.2	703.7
Peanut	6.42	–3.35	72.2	406.9	4.9	700.7
Pecan	6.03	–2.16	73.1	288.9	0.0	602.8
Pinenut	6.42	–5.35	15.0	550.0	4.0	690.0
Pistachio, salted	–35.80	–3.70	130.0	500.0	390.0	1100.0
Pumpkin seed, salted	–14.40	–10.56	44.0	1100.0	190.0	840.0
Sesame seed, hulled	–1.18	–5.68	162.0	730.0	24.0	170.0
Sesame seed, unhulled	0.05	5.44	1160.0	616.0	60.0	725.0
Sunflower seed	5.60	–7.17	120.0	837.0	30.0	920.0
Walnut	4.26	–2.81	99.0	380.0	2.0	450.0
Seafood						
Flounder	–5.95	–1.83	11.9	195.4	78.1	342.4
Hijiki seaweed	–124.00	13.00	1400.0	100.0	1400.0	4400.0
Kombu kelp	–308.11	8.53	1093.0	240.0	3007.0	5273.0

Food	Residues (mg/g)		Mineral amounts (mg/100 g)			
	K-res	Ca-res	Ca	P	Na	K
Nori sheets	8.40	−2.00	410.0	610.0	130.0	2400.0
Salmon, tinned	−42.81	−0.90	195.9	285.9	386.8	360.9
Sardine, tinned	−93.89	−0.61	442.9	503.6	832.1	596.4
Schnapper	−4.82	−1.98	16.1	214.3	67.1	323.4
Trout	−5.10	−2.15	25.0	240.0	75.0	390.0
Tuna	−2.13	−1.74	16.0	190.0	41.0	279.0
Sugars						
Honey	−0.05	0.00	4.8	4.8	4.8	52.4
Sugar, brown	−0.16	0.66	85.0	19.1	30.0	344.1
Sugar, white	−0.09	0.00	0.0	0.0	1.0	3.0
Vegetables						
Artichoke	3.84	−0.52	26.0	78.0	3.0	420.0
Asparagus	2.51	−0.40	22.2	62.2	2.2	277.8
Bamboo shoot	5.66	−0.49	13.8	63.0	0.0	566.4
Beet green	−9.90	0.79	119.0	40.0	130.0	570.0
Beetroot	−3.85	−0.17	16.3	33.3	60.0	334.8
Bok choy	1.78	−0.11	25.0	36.0	6.0	250.0
Broccoli	2.02	0.25	103.0	78.0	15.0	382.0
Brussels sprout	2.22	−0.44	36.0	80.0	14.0	390.0
Cabbage	−0.07	0.20	48.6	28.6	20.0	232.9
Carrot	−2.23	0.01	37.0	36.0	47.0	341.0
Carrot juice	−2.17	−0.32	3.7	35.7	46.3	337.9
Cauliflower	1.39	−0.31	25.0	56.0	13.0	295.0
Celery	−11.69	0.11	39.2	28.3	125.8	340.8
Chard (silverbeet)	−12.14	0.49	88.0	39.0	147.0	550.0
Chilli, green	1.38	−0.09	4.9	13.9	4.2	188.6
Chinese (white) cabbage	1.40	−0.11	60.0	71.0	10.0	260.0
Chive	2.50	0.30	70.0	40.0	0.0	250.0
Collard	−1.15	1.40	203.0	63.0	43.0	401.0
Cress	4.90	0.00	80.0	80.0	10.0	610.0
Cucumber	0.91	−0.02	24.8	26.7	5.7	160.0
Dandelion green	−5.15	1.21	187.0	66.0	76.0	397.0
Dock (sorrel)	2.78	0.25	66.0	41.0	5.0	338.0

Food	Residues (mg/g)		Mineral amounts (mg/100 g)			
	K-res	Ca-res	Ca	P	Na	K
Eggplant	1.90	−0.14	12.0	26.0	2.0	214.0
Endive	1.26	0.28	82.0	54.0	14.0	294.0
Gai choy	0.20	1.30	180.0	50.0	30.0	380.0
Garlic	1.33	−1.67	33.3	200.0	33.3	533.3
Ginger	1.92	−0.13	23.0	36.0	6.0	264.0
Green pepper (capsicum)	0.63	−0.14	8.8	22.5	12.5	212.5
Kale	−5.82	1.06	179.0	73.0	75.0	318.0
Kohlrabi	2.76	−0.09	40.7	50.0	8.0	372.0
Leek	2.87	0.02	52.0	50.0	5.0	347.0
Lettuce, leaf	1.55	0.42	67.3	25.5	9.1	263.6
Mushroom	2.26	−1.10	5.7	115.7	15.7	414.3
Mustard green	−0.07	1.33	183.0	50.0	32.0	377.0
Okra	2.13	0.41	92.0	51.0	3.0	249.0
Onion	0.37	−0.09	27.1	35.9	10.0	157.1
Parsley	1.87	1.40	203.3	63.3	45.0	726.7
Parsnip	3.97	−0.27	50.0	77.0	12.0	541.0
Pea	2.91	−0.90	26.2	115.9	2.1	315.9
Potato	3.67	−0.46	7.3	53.3	3.3	407.3
Potato, french fries + salt	−21.80	−0.77	9.0	86.0	236.0	652.0
Pumpkin	2.16	−0.01	24.9	26.1	2.0	240.0
Radish	0.98	0.00	28.0	28.0	16.0	290.0
Scallion (spring onion)	1.71	0.12	51.0	39.0	5.0	231.0
Shallot	2.10	−0.20	40.0	60.0	10.0	330.0
Spinach	−3.80	0.42	92.7	50.9	70.9	470.9
Squash, summer (zucchini)	1.90	−0.01	28.0	29.0	1.0	202.0
Squash, winter	3.72	0.08	31.0	23.0	1.0	384.0
Sum choy (Na est.)	−1.03	1.09	144.0	35.0	30.0	257.0
Sweet potato	1.19	−0.14	31.5	45.2	9.6	234.2
Tomato	2.12	−0.13	13.3	26.7	2.7	244.0
Turnip	−3.23	0.09	39.2	30.0	49.2	267.7
Turnip green	3.20	1.88	246.0	58.0	10.0	440.0
Watercress	−3.34	0.97	151.4	54.3	51.4	282.9

Epilogue

T he exploration of the realm of CaPNaK is ongoing. If you wish to play a part in the process, please respond to the questionnaire on p. 185. Alternatively, if you would like to be informed about new developments and opportunities, send your name and address to me at the address given.

I hope many of you reading this book will be convinced that symbiotic eating with fruit as the predominant staple is your best choice. Persisting in changing to this way of eating is difficult, and I hope this book has equipped you to avoid the pitfalls. Others will agree only in part, or be unwilling to diverge so far from the main-stream madness.

If you now agree with the symbiotic way of eating, then cultivate your inner strength to live by this ideal. However, do not cling to it too dogmatically—your freedom and love are even higher ideals.

Now it is your time to consider what changes you can and will make to move in the direction of eco-eating. Take a moment now to plan your changes. Even the smallest change is worthwhile for you, us all, and the planet.

References

Aihara, H. 1982. *Acid and Alkaline*. Rev. edn. Georges Ohsawa Macrobiotic Foundation, Oroville, Calif.

Asahi Shimbun Japan Almanac 1993. Asahi Shimbun Publishing Co., Tokyo.

Australian Institute of Health 1994. *Australian Health*. AGPS, Canberra.

Barzel, U. S. 1982. 'Acid Loading and Osteoporosis'. *J. Amer. Geriatrics Soc.* vol. 30, no. 9, Sept. 1982.

Berger, S. M. 1985. *Dr. Berger's Immune Power Diet*. New American Library, New York.

Bronner, F. & Comar, C. L. (eds) 1960. *Mineral Metabolism: An Advanced Treatise*. Academic Press, New York.

Brook, S. 1987. A Physical Theory of Organization and Consequent Neural Model of Spatio-temporal Pattern Acquisition. MSc thesis, School of Architecture and Engineering, Deakin University, Geelong, Vic.

Colbin, A. 1986. *Food and Healing*. Ballantine Books, New York.

Diamond, H. & Diamond M. 1985. *Fit for Life*. Warner Books, New York.

Draper, H. H., Scythes, C. A. 1981. 'Calcium, phosphorus and osteoporosis'. *Federation Proc.* 40 (9): 2434–38.

Dunbar, R. 1991. 'Foraging for nature's balanced diet'. *New Scientist*, vol. 131, no. 1784, pp. 21–4, 31 August.

EarthSave Foundation 1992. *Our Food, Our World*, EarthSave Foundation, Santa Cruz, Calif.

Ehret, A. 1953. *Mucusless Diet Healing System*. Ehret Literature Publishing Company, Beaumont, Calif. [published posthumously].

Gasser, C. S. & Fraley, R. T. 1992. 'Transgenic crops'. *Scientific American*, vol. 226, no. 6, p. 34, June.

Goulder, L. & Lutwak, L. 1988. *The Strong Bones Diet*. Triad Publishing Company, Gainesville, Fla.

Guyton, A. C. 1977. *Basic Human Physiology*. W. B. Saunders Company, Philadelphia, Penn.

Haas, R. 1983. *Eat to Win*. Penguin, New York.

Hewitt, J. 1964. *About Seafoods*. Thursons, London.

Horne, R. 1985. *The Health Revolution*. 4th edn. Happy Landings, Avalon Beach, NSW.

Jung, C. G. 1971. *Psychological Types*. Routledge & Kegan Paul, London.

Kenton, L, & Kenton, S. 1984. *Raw Energy: Eat Your Way to Radiant Health*. Century Arrow, London.

Kincaid-Smith, P. 1983. *Textbook of Clinical Medicine*. ADIS Health Science Press, Sydney.

Kulvinskas, V. 1975. *Survival into the 21st Century*. Omangod Press, Wethersfield, Conn.

Langley, G. 1988. *Vegan Nutrition*. Vegan Society, East Sussex, UK.

Lappe, F. M. 1975. *Diet for a Small Planet*. Ballantine Books, New York.

Milton, K. 1993. 'Diet and primate evolution'. *Scientific American*, vol. 269, p. 71, August 1993.

Mulham, M. (1995). 'Releasing Fat'. *Australian Wellbeing*, no. 58, pp. 60–5.

National Health and Medical Research Council 1991. *Recommended Dietary Intakes for Use in Australia*. AGPS, Canberra.

Nutrition Search Inc. 1979. *Nutrition Almanac*. McGraw-Hill, New York.

Pearson, D. & Shaw, S. 1982. *Life Extension*. Warner Books, New York.

Pritikin, N. with McGrady, P. Jr 1973. *The Pritikin Program for Diet and Exercise*. Grosset & Dunlap, New York.

Rensberger, B. 'Teeth Show Fruit Was the Staple'. *New York Times*, p. C1, 15 May.

Robbins, J. (1987). *Diet for a New America*. Stillpoint Publishing, Walpole, New Hamps., p. 193.

Santillo, H. 1987. *Food Enzymes: The Key to Radiant Health*. Hohm Press, Prescott Valley, Ariz.

Thomas, P. R. (ed.) 1991. *Improving America's Diet and Health*. National Academy Press, Washington, DC.

Truswell, A. S. 1992. 'ABC of Nutrition'. *British Medical Journal*. [monograph].

United States Department of Agriculture 1990. 'Composition of Foods', in *Agriculture Handbook*, No. 8, USDA, Washington, DC.

United States Department of Health and Human Services 1990. *Healthy People 2000: National Health Promotion and Disease Prevention Objectives.* USDHHS, Washington, DC.

Walker, N. 1949. *Become Younger.* O'Sullivan Woodside & Company, Phoenix, Ariz.

Waterhouse, D. 1993. *Outsmarting the Female Fat Cell.* Hodder & Stoughton, London.

Index

acid:
   fruit category 57
   Macrobiotic 2
   phosphorus 22, 80, 81, 141, 168
   state 43, 79, 129, 151
   see also CaPNaK; food
acne 9, 111
addictions 97, 98, 103, 105, 112, 117, 140
   caffeine 9, 106, 111, 122
agriculture:
   and diet 30, 61, 138, 141, 144, 145, 146
   see also permaculture
alkaline:
   Macrobiotic 2
   state 32, 43, 74, 116, 139, 140, 151,
      168
   see also CaPNaK; food; Macrobiotic
      diet
allergies 68, 70, 94
antioxidants *see* free radicals

beauty 78, 111, 112
bingeing 70, 74, 131
blood test 89
blood-sugar level 24, 98, 105, 120, 123,
   126, 129, 130
body fluids 46, 82, 107, 135, 160
body-mind 22, 23, 43, 45, 80, 74, 98,
   165, 168, 170
bones:
   problems 12, 30, 36, 37, 43, 76, 79,
      81, 87
   see also calcium
brain function 52, 62, 128, 129, 134

caffeine *see* addictions
calcium:
   deficiency 11, 12, 25, 36, 39, 73, 79,
      87; *see also* phosphorus, excess
   excess 39; *see also* phosphorus,
      deficiency
   intake 38, 44, 74, 139, 162
   sources 11, 12, 40, 42, 107
   see also bones; CaPNaK
cancer:
   and immunity 67
   from meat 9, 68, 144
   prevention 87, 109, 144
CapNaK:
   balance, 11, 16, 23, 45, 46, 58, 59,
      89, 92, 93, 103, 151, 160, 163, 165
   chart 1, 3, 11, 15, 17, 18, 19, 20, 21,
      22, 24, 40, 75, 79, 82, 84, 91, 92,
      93, 94, 98, 116, 133, 138, 160,
      162, 163, 164, 165, 166, 184
   complementary effects 18, 20, 21,
      133, 151, 168
   overdose symptoms 19, 39, 46
carbohydrates:
   complex 101
   fruit 25, 49, 58, 98
cardiovascular disease 8, 71, 81, 144
cereal *see* grain
chakras:
   food 32, 33, 131
   psychophysical 35, 95, 96
children, and food 136, 137
cholesterol 8, 71, 89, 109
climate, and diet 91, 94

coldness 18, 46, 82, 84, 91, 93, 142
cooking:
   enzyme destruction 9, 53
   see also food, mutilation
craving *see* additions

dairy foods:
   and cardiovascular disease 8
   and osteoporosis 37, 79
   problems 41, 62, 66, 69, 74, 137
debauchery, conscious 97
dieting 77
   see also diets
diets *see* agriculture and diet; climate
   and diet; digestion; emotional
   problems; fasting; fat; grain-based
   diet; hominid diet; live-food diet;
   Macrobiotic diet; meat-based diet;
   menu, daily; oil; primate diet;
   Pritikin diet; symbiotic diet; vegan
   diet; vegetarian diet
digestion 10, 35, 51, 116, 121, 123
   enzymes 53, 139
   fibre 29
   fruit 24, 123, 138
   problems 41, 49, 53

ecome 114, 142
emotions:
   personality types 133, 134
   problems 60, 70, 75, 100, 111, 115,
     124, 130, 140
energy from food 49, 99, 120, 125, 136
enlivenment, definition 34, 132
environment, destruction of 119, 129,
    138, 141, 144, 146
enzymes:
   free radicals 88
   in fruit 24, 53, 67
   maximum 9, 137
exercise:
   and health 72, 76, 125, 126, 137
   load-bearing 43
eyes 111, 112

fasting 126
fat:
   gain 12, 79, 137
   loss 25, 74
   over-fat 38, 68, 74, 135
   problems 49, 50, 71, 74
   rancid 71, 80, 88
   types 63, 72, 80, 88
   under-fat 10, 38, 100
fibre, digestion of 29
fish 7, 13, 62
   see also herbo-pisco-fruitarian
fitness 10, 89, 126
   see also exercise
fluids *see* body fluids
food:
   acid-forming 12
   alkali-forming 12
   combining 21, 52, 56, 57, 101, 151
   composition 24, 170
   groups 23
   and happiness 98
   log 32
   mutilation 30, 31, 66, 85, 101, 107,
     120, 130, 138, 142
   spiritual 95, 97, 148
   see also chakras; children; energy
     from food; exercise
free radicals 71, 87, 127
fruit:
   benefits 24, 142
   dried 99, 124, 139
   and refrigeration 94, 142
   sugar 2, 24, 123, 129, 140
fruitarian:
   diet 1, 10, 25, 28, 30, 41, 117, 138
   ideadlism 13, 41, 61, 81, 86
   network 2, 13
   yin 26
   see also grain, and fruit; herbo-
     fruitarian; herbo-pisco-fruitarian

gas 2, 10, 58
grain, and fruit 2, 3, 27, 81, 159

grain-based diet 8, 27, 36, 49, 63, 67,
    69, 86, 98, 159
  see also grain, and fruit; Macrobiotic
    diet
grazing *see* hunger

headache:
  from caffeine 9
  see also CaPNaK, overdose
    symptoms; sodium, deficiency
health, poor 8, 72, 74
  see also cardiovascular disease
heart disease *see* cardiovascular
    disease
herbo-fruitarian 11, 27, 29, 86
herbo-pisco-fruitarian 27, 52, 81
hominid diet 29
Horne, Ross 9, 136
hot, feeling 18, 46, 82, 84, 121
hunger, and grazing 52, 59, 123, 139
hunting 30, 67
hyperactive state 81
hypoglycaemia *see* blood-sugar
    level

immunity:
  effectiveness 60, 66, 146
  enzymes 53, 67, 139
  infection, from water 10, 108

juices 87, 99, 124, 126, 151, 153

Kulvinskas, Viktoras 10, 11

live-food diet 1, 28, 54, 67, 101, 107,
    111, 130
longevity:
  dietary strategies 86
  enzymes 55, 137
love, spiritual 95, 148

Macrobiotic diet 1, 2, 47, 63, 90, 104
  see also grain-based diet
mango, how to eat 83, 113

meat-based diet 8, 52, 67, 100, 115,
    142, 144, 146
  see also hunting

meditation:
  forms 35
  and stress 9, 95, 116
  see also stress
menopause *see* bones
menstruation, irregular 136
menu, daily 26, 50, 76, 85, 88, 94, 99,
    107, 151
metabolism, changing 76
minerals:
  deficiencies 60, 63, 106
  iron 60
  overdose 23, 63
  residue 16, 21, 160, 168, 170
  zinc 26, 135
money saving 94, 95, 119
mucus 41
muscle power 125, 127, 129
mutilation *see* food, mutilation

nuts, intake 80, 78, 108, 138, 159

oil 24, 50, 80, 88
organic food 61, 138, 141
  see also agriculture
organisation, in nature 31
osteoporosis *see* bones
overdose symptoms *see* CaPNaK

permaculture 145
  see also agriculture
personality *see* emotions
phosphorus:
  deficiency 39; see also calcium,
    excess
  excess 36, 39, 63, 85, 122, 141, 162;
    see also calcium, deficiency
  fat loss 75
  sources 11
  see also CaPNaK

positive effects *see* CaPNaK

potassium:

  balancing 11, 46, 47, 58, 103

  deficiency 46; *see also* sodium, excess

  excess 46; *see also* sodium, deficiency

  sources 84

  see also CaPNaK

pregnancy *see* women

primate diet 29, 52, 66, 135

Pritikin diet 1, 26, 72, 86

problems *see* addictions; bingeing;
      bones; dairy foods; diet;
      digestion; fat; menstruation;
      sleeping; smoking; stress; sugar;
      teeth; toxins

protein:

  complete 25

  excess 36, 40, 49, 126, 127, 137, 158

  sources 25, 26, 137

recipes, live-food preparation 151

seaweed 63, 82, 135

seeds *see* nuts

sex:

  libido 27, 135

  spiritual 95

skin 9, 83, 85, 88, 109, 111, 124, 144

sleeping 123

smoking 105, 112, 124

social eating 100, 115, 119, 129, 131,
      138, 140, 141, 144, 146

sodium:

  deficiency 26, 45, 46, 58, 84, 99,
      108, 135, 162; *see also* potassium,
      excess

  excess 39, 45, 46, 126; *see also*
      potassium, deficiency

  sources 11, 45, 83, 108

  see also CaPNaK

sport, 125, 126

  see also exercise

stress 124, 131, 136, 137

  see also meditation

sugar:

  problems 9, 24, 70, 105, 130

  see also fruit

supplements 12, 59, 63

symbiotic diet 1, 26, 28, 50, 63, 117,
      119, 124, 142, 162

symbiotic evolution 66, 93, 146

symbiotic transition 28, 100, 130, 145,
      177, 184

symptoms *see* CaPNaK

taste treats 101, 103, 138, 151

  see also recipes

teeth 10, 12, 29, 73

toxins, elimination 13, 66, 69, 78, 109,
      136, 137, 145

vegan diet 1, 13, 34, 35, 90, 159

vegetables, green-leaf 12, 41, 42, 63,
      108, 112, 138

vegetarian diet 1, 93

vitamins:

  deficiencies 60

  vitamin A 60

  vitamin B 49, 60, 61, 106, 124

  vitamin B_{12} 7, 13, 27, 62, 138, 159

  vitamin C 60, 88, 107

  vitamin D 109, 124

  vitamin E 88

Walker, Norman 87

water, drinking 10, 25, 59, 83, 90, 107,
      108, 121, 126, 144

weight *see* fat

women:

  and nutrition 61, 78, 135

  pregnancy 41, 63, 136, 137, 140

  see also bones; menstruation

work 120, 123

yang:

  definition 47, 48

  and emotions 131

  Macrobiotic 2

yin:

  definition 47, 48

  and emotions 116, 124, 131

  Macrobiotic 2, 104

Questionnaire

I wish to establish a qualitative databank of the experiences of people resulting from this book. I also wish to maintain contact with people affected by this book to provide the opportunity for medical research in the future.

If you are interested, please complete the following, and send to my address on the next page:

Briefly describe your lifestyle.

Describe your diet before reading this book (include food log, if possible).

Describe your diet after reading this book (include food log, if possible).

Describe any states of your body-mind affected after changing to eco-eating.

Describe any unhealthy states of your body-mind not affected after changing to eco–eating.

What is your date of birth?

Are you male or female?

Which area of the world do you live in?

If you wish to be kept informed, please include your name and address.

Are you interested in computer software that will calculate your cumulative CaPNaK mineral residues?

Training Consultation

You can experience and learn the art of symbiotic eating at my live-in seminars or at a seminar in your area. You will be guided through the practicalities of eating live foods and using the CaPNaK Chart to fine-tune your health.

Symbiotic lifestyle training sessions are held at my home in an ocean-forest community on the mid-north coast of NSW. You can experience a solar-permaculture-based lifestyle in my ecome (ecological home), and take a ride in my solar vehicle. You will have time to reflect and create meaningful change in your life in relation to nurturing the Earth.

Please apply in writing.

Colour Poster

The CaPNaK Chart will help you in the following ways:
- enable you to rebalance your disturbances before they grow into diseases
- empower you to adjust your physical and mental states to suit your needs
- help you to easily identify foods by their picture
- provide a handy reference on your wall
- act as a decorative and colourful aid for discussion with your friends
- show all of the foods on one large chart, allowing you to select balancing foods at a glance.

If you wish to order a copy of the colour poster of this chart (38 cm × 54 cm; $9.75 each) please write to:

Sapoty Brook (CaPNaK)
PO Box 8
REPTON NSW 2454

Include your payment and postal address.